MILADY'S STANDARD

COSMETOLOGY STUDY GUIDE:

THE ESSENTIAL COMPANION

MILADY'S STANDARD

COSMETOLOGY STUDY GUIDE:

THE ESSENTIAL COMPANION

Letha Barnes

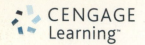
CENGAGE
Learning™

**Milady's Standard: Cosmetology Study Guide:
The Essential Companion**
Letha Barnes

For product information and technology assistance, contact us at
Cengage Learning Customer & Sales Support, 1-800-354-9706

For permission to use material from this text or product,
submit all requests online at **cengage.com/permissions**
Further permissions questions can be emailed to
permissionrequest@cengage.com

ISBN-13: 978-1-4180-4940-9

ISBN-10: 1-4180-4940-9

Milady
Executive Woods
5 Maxwell Drive
Clifton Park, NY 12065
USA

Cengage Learning is a leading provider of customized learning solutions with office locations around the globe, including Singapore, the United Kingdom, Australia, Mexico, Brazil, and Japan. Locate your local office at:
international.cengage.com/region

Cengage Learning products are represented in Canada by Nelson Education, Ltd.

For your lifelong learning solutions, visit **delmar.cengage.com**

Visit our corporate website at **www.cengage.com**

Notice to the Reader
Publisher does not warrant or guarantee any of the products described herein or perform any independent analysis in connection with any of the product information contained herein. Publisher does not assume, and expressly disclaims, any obligation to obtain and include information other than that provided to it by the manufacturer. The reader is expressly warned to consider and adopt all safety precautions that might be indicated by the activities described herein and to avoid all potential hazards. By following the instructions contained herein, the reader willingly assumes all risks in connection with such instructions. The publisher makes no representations or warranties of any kind, including but not limited to, the warranties of fitness for particular purpose or merchantability, nor are any such representations implied with respect to the material set forth herein, and the publisher takes no responsibility with respect to such material. The publisher shall not be liable for any special, consequential, or exemplary damages resulting, in whole or part, from the readers' use of, or reliance upon, this material.

Printed in the United States of America
10 11

CONTENTS

PREFACE xv

CHAPTER 1
HISTORY & CAREER OPPORTUNITIES 1
Essential Objectives 1
Essential History and Opportunities: Why is knowing about this history and evolution of this industry so important to my success in cosmetology or a related field? 2
Essential Concepts: What are the essentials about the industry's history and the career opportunities available? 3
Essential Experience 1
   Historical Time Line 4
Essential Experience 2
   Mind Mapping 6
Essential Experience 3
   Character Study and Report 7
Essential Experience 4
   Word Scramble 8
Essential Review 9
Essential Discoveries
and Accomplishments 11

CHAPTER 2
LIFE SKILLS 12
Essential Objectives 12
Essential Life Skills: Why do I need to learn about life skills in order to be successful as a cosmetologist? 13
Essential Concepts of Life Skills Management: What do I need to know about life skills management in order to be effective as a licensed professional? 14
Essential Experience 1
   Goals Setting 15
Essential Experience 2
   Collage of Goals 16
Essential Experience 3
   Mind Map of Yourself Today 17
Essential Experience 4
   Mind Map Your Future 18

Essential Experience 5
   Track Your Attendance 19
Essential Experience 6
Self-Assessment of Personal
Characteristics 20
Essential Experience 7
   Time Management 21
Essential Experience 8
   Action Plan for Time Management 23
Essential Experience 9
   Is Your Bad Attitude an Addiction? 24
Essential Review 26
Essential Discoveries
and Accomplishments 28

CHAPTER 3
YOUR PROFESSIONAL IMAGE 29
Essential Objectives 29
Essential Professionalism: Why are professionalism and my image so important to my success in cosmetology or a related field? 30
Essential Concepts: What are the essentials about image and professional development? 31
Essential Experience 1
   What Does Your Professional Image
   Say About You? 32
Essential Experience 2
   Policy Development 33
Essential Experience 3
   Word Scramble—
   Your Professional Image 34
Essential Experience 4
   Rate Your Image 35
Essential Experience 5
   Analyze Your Personal Lifestyle 36
Essential Experience 6
   Your Attitude—
   What Does It Say About You? 37
Essential Review 38
Essential Discoveries
and Accomplishments 39

CHAPTER 4

COMMUNICATING FOR SUCCESS 40

Essential Objectives.................................. 40
Essential Communication Skills: Why do I need to learn about communicating when I just want to cut hair?.......................... 41
Essential Concepts for Communicating Effectively: What do I need to know about communicating for success in order to provide quality service to my clients and enjoy career success?........................ 42
Essential Experience 1
    Body Language Matching Exercise...... 43
Essential Experience 2
    Eye Movement 44
Essential Experience 3
    Mind Map Consultation Interference 45
Essential Experience 4
    Partner Messaging 46
Essential Experience 5
    Role-Playing a Dissatisfied Client....... 47
Essential Experience 6
    Windowpane—
    Client Consultation Tools 48
Essential Experience 7
    Topics to Avoid 49
Essential Review 50
Essential Discoveries and Accomplishments 52

CHAPTER 5

INFECTION CONTROL: PRINCIPLES & PRACTICES 53

Essential Objectives.................................. 53
Essential Principles and Practices of Infection Control: Why do I need to know about the principles of infection control?.................. 54
Essential Concepts: What are the essential concepts of providing the safest possible environment using effective decontamination and infection control procedures?.............. 55
Essential Experience 1
    Mind Mapping.............................. 56

Essential Experience 2 57
Essential Experience 3 58
Essential Experience 4
    Word Scramble—Bacteriology 59
Essential Experience 5 61
Essential Experience 6 63
Essential Experience 7
    Word Search—Decontamination 65
Essential Review 66
Essential Discoveries and Accomplishments 69

CHAPTER 6

GENERAL ANATOMY AND PHYSIOLOGY 70

Essential Objectives.................................. 70
Essential Anatomy and Physiology: Why do I need to know about cells and the anatomy and physiology of the body when I just want to do hair?.................................... 71
Essential Concepts: What do I need to learn about cells and anatomy and physiology to be more effective as a cosmetologist?........ 72
Essential Experience 1
    Mind Map—Cell Development............ 73
Essential Experience 2
    Organs 74
Essential Experience 3
    Matching Exercise—Body Systems 75
Essential Experience 4
    Matching Exercise A—
    The Muscular System 76
Essential Experience 5
    Matching Exercise B—
    The Muscular System 77
Essential Experience 6
    Bones and Muscles of the Cranium 78
Essential Experience 7
    Word Search A—Circulatory System.... 79
Essential Experience 8
    Word Search B—Circulatory System....80
Essential Review 81
Essential Discoveries and Accomplishments 87

CHAPTER 7

SKIN STRUCTURE & GROWTH 88

Essential Objectives................................88
Essential Histology of the Skin: Why do I
need to learn about the skin structure and
growth when I really want to specialize
as a hair designer?................................89
Essential Concepts: What do I need to know
about the structure and growth of the skin
in order to perform professionally as a
cosmetologist?................................90
Essential Experience 1
  Analysis of the Epidermis 91
Essential Experience 2
  Skin Layer Reconstruction 92
Essential Experience 3
  Matching 93
Essential Experience 4
  Crossword Puzzle........................94
Essential Review................................95
Essential Discoveries
and Accomplishments..........................98

CHAPTER 8

NAIL STRUCTURE & GROWTH 99

Essential Objectives................................99
Essential Nail Structure and Growth: I am
going to be a cosmetologist; why do I need
to learn about the structure of the nail?.....100
Essential Concepts of Nail Structure and
Growth, Diseases, and Disorders: What do I
need to know about the nail, its structure,
and growth in order to provide quality
manicuring and pedicuring services?........101
Essential Experience 1 102
Essential Experience 2
  Matching Exercise—Structures
  Surrounding the Nail....................103
Essential Experience 3
  Windowpane 104
Essential Experience 4
  Word Search 105

Essential Review................................106
Essential Discoveries
and Accomplishments..........................108

CHAPTER 9

PROPERTIES OF THE HAIR & SCALP 109

Essential Objectives..........................109
Essential Properties of the Hair and Scalp:
How will knowing about the underlying theory of
the properties of the hair and scalp help me
to be a more successful cosmetologist? 110
Essential Concepts: What are the key
concepts a professional cosmetologist must
understand in order to properly analyze
a client's hair and prescribe appropriate
corrective treatments?..........................111
Essential Experience 1
  Hair Purpose 112
Essential Experience 2
  Hair Follicle Structure 113
Essential Experience 3
  Hair Structure..........................114
Essential Experience 4
  Hair Replacement and Growth 115
Essential Experience 5
  Directional Hair Growth................116
Essential Experience 6
  Word Search—
  Properties of the Hair and Scalp.......117
Essential Experience 7
  Crossword Puzzle—
  Properties of the Hair and Scalp.......119
Essential Experience 8
  Grouping Properties of the Hair
  and Scalp by Category..................121
Essential Review................................122
Essential Discoveries
and Accomplishments..........................126

CHAPTER 10

THE BASICS OF CHEMISTRY 127

Essential Objectives 127
Essential Chemistry: Why is a basic
knowledge of chemistry important to
my career as a cosmetologist? 128
Essential Concepts: What do I need to
know about basic chemistry in order to
be successful and more effective as a
professional cosmetologist? 129
Essential Experience 1
    Organic Versus Inorganic Chemistry 130
Essential Experience 2
    Product Research 131
Essential Experience 3
    Matter 132
Essential Experience 4
    Elements 133
Essential Experience 5
    Litmus Paper Testing 134
Essential Experience 6
    Crossword Puzzle 135
Essential Experience 7
    Word Search 136
Essential Experience 8
    Matching Exercise 138
Essential Review 139
Essential Discoveries
and Accomplishments 141

CHAPTER 11

THE BASICS OF ELECTRICITY 142

Essential Objectives 142
Essential Electricity: Why is a basic
knowledge of electricity important to
my career as a cosmetologist? 143
Essential Concepts: What do I need to
know about basic electricity in order to
be successful and more effective as a
professional cosmetologist? 144

Essential Experience 1
    Matching Exercise—Electrical
    Measurements 145
Essential Experience 2
    Safety of Electrical Equipment 146
Essential Experience 3
    Crossword Puzzle—Electricity 147
Essential Experience 4
    Word Scramble—Electricity 148
Essential Experience 5
    The Visible Spectrum 149
Essential Review 150
Essential Discoveries
and Accomplishments 152

CHAPTER 12

PRINCIPLES OF HAIR DESIGN 153

Essential Objectives 153
Essential Design in Hairstyling: Why is
understanding the basic elements of
design so important to my success as a
cosmetologist? 154
Essential Concepts: If there are so many
key "ingredients" to hair design, where
do I begin? 155
Essential Experience 1
    The Elements of Design 156
Essential Experience 2
    The Principles of Design 160
Essential Experience 3
    Windowpane—Facial Types 164
Essential Experience 4
    Special Considerations A 165
    Special Considerations B 166
Essential Experience 5
    Crossword Puzzle—
    Design in Hairstyling 167
Essential Review 168
Essential Discoveries
and Accomplishments 173

CHAPTER 13
SHAMPOOING, RINSING, AND CONDITIONING 174

Essential Objectives............................. 174
Essential Shampooing and Conditioning: Why are shampooing and conditioning so important to my training when they seem to be such insignificant services? 175
Essential Concepts: What do I need to know about shampooing, rinsing, and conditioning in order to provide a quality service? 176
Essential Experience 1 177
Essential Experience 2 178
Essential Experience 3 179
Essential Experience 4 180
Essential Experience 5 181
Essential Experience 6
   Crossword Puzzle—Shampooing, Rinsing, and Conditioning 182
Essential Rubrics 183
Essential Review 185
Essential Discoveries and Accomplishments 187

CHAPTER 14
HAIRCUTTING 188

Essential Objectives............................. 188
Essential Haircutting: I really want to specialize in hair design, so why is it so important for me to master the art of haircutting? 189
Essential Concepts: What are the most important techniques and procedures I should learn to become a good haircutter? 190
Essential Experience 1
   Identify the Tools......................... 191
Essential Experience 2
   Windowpane 192
Essential Experience 3
   Terms...................................... 193
Essential Experience 4 195

Essential Experience 5 196
Essential Experience 6
   Word Scramble............................ 197
Essential Experience 7
   Word Search—Haircutting 198
Essential Experience 8 199
Essential Experience 9
   Word Search 200
Essential Rubrics 201
Essential Review 207
Essential Discoveries and Accomplishments 210

CHAPTER 15
HAIRSTYLING 211

Essential Objectives............................. 211
Essential Wet Hairstyling: What roles will wet hairstyling, thermal hairstyling, and hair pressing play in my success as a cosmetologist?................................. 212
Essential Wet Hairstyling Concepts: What are the most important elements in hairstyling that I need to know?............. 214
Essential Experience 1
   Mind Map of Wet Hairstyling 215
Essential Experience 2
   Windowpane—Pin Curls 216
Essential Experience 3
   Pin Curl Shaping and Bases............ 217
Essential Experience 4
   Windowpane—Roller Placement 218
Essential Experience 5
   Word Search 219
Essential Experience 6
   Iron Manipulations....................... 221
Essential Experience 7
   Safety Precautions 222
Essential Experience 8
   Thermal Curling Preparation 223
Essential Experience 9
   Windowpaning—Thermal Curling 224
Essential Experience 10
   Thermal Waving With Conventional Thermal Irons 225

Essential Experience 11
Types of Hair Pressing.................... 228
Essential Experience 12
Product Knowledge...................... 229
Essential Experience 13
Hair and Scalp Analysis 230
Essential Experience 14
Jeopardy 231
Essential Rubrics 233
Essential Review 239
Essential Discoveries
and Accomplishments 247

CHAPTER 16

BRAIDING & BRAID EXTENSIONS 248
Essential Objectives............................... 248
Essential Braiding: Why do I need to learn
about braiding when I am not interested
in providing these services? 249
Essential Concepts: What do I need to
know about braiding in order to provide
a quality service?................................. 250
Essential Experience 1
Preparing Textured Hair
for Braiding 251
Essential Experience 2
The Developmental Stages
of Locks 252
Essential Experience 3
Procedure for Basic Cornrows 253
Essential Experience 4
Word Search 255
Essential Experience 5
Research and Design...................... 257
Essential Rubrics 258
Essential Review 261
Essential Discoveries
and Accomplishments 265

CHAPTER 17

WIGS & HAIR ENHANCEMENTS............266
Essential Objectives............................... 266
Essential Aspects of Wigs and Hair
Enhancements: Do people really still
wear wigs, and why should I know how
to handle them?................................. 267
Essential Concepts: What can really be so
hard about handling wigs, and what do I
really need to know? 268
Essential Experience 1
The History of Wigs 269
Essential Experience 2
Wig Measurements........................ 270
Essential Experience 3
Matching Exercise 271
Essential Experience 4
Crossword Puzzle.......................... 272
Essential Experience 5
Windowpane—Wig Care.................. 273
Essential Review............................... 274
Essential Discoveries
and Accomplishments 276

CHAPTER 18

CHEMICAL TEXTURE SERVICES.............277
Essential Objectives............................... 277
Essential Chemical Texture Services: What
role will permanent waving and hair
relaxing have in my career when all I
really want to do is style hair? 278
Essential Concepts: Exactly what am I going
to need to learn about permanent waving
and chemical hair relaxing to be considered
competent in this particular skill?.............. 279
Essential Experience 1
Defining Permanent Waving
and Identifying Textures................ 280
Essential Experience 2
Hair Analysis 281

Essential Experience 3
    Product Research 281
Essential Experience 4
    Matching 282
Essential Experience 5
    Product Research 283
Essential Experience 6
    Purpose and Action of Chemical
    Hair Relaxing 284
Essential Experience 7
    Word Search—Chemical
    Texture Services 286
Essential Rubrics 288
Essential Review 296
*Essential Discoveries
and Accomplishments* 307

CHAPTER 19

HAIRCOLORING 308

Essential Objectives 308
*Essential Haircoloring: Will I get over my
fear of haircolor and be able to formulate
and apply it successfully in the salon?* 309
*Essential Concepts: What are the key
concepts or elements in haircoloring
that I need to know to be successful?* 310
Essential Experience 1
    The Color Wheel 311
Essential Experience 2
    Haircolor Challenges/Corrective
    Solutions 312
Essential Experience 3
    The Level System 313
Essential Experience 4
    The Four Classifications of Color 314
Essential Experience 5
    Windowpane—Color Applications..... 315
Essential Experience 6
    Crossword Puzzle—Haircolor 316
Essential Experience 7
    Word Search—Haircolor 317
Essential Experience 8
    Matching Exercise—Haircolor.......... 319

Essential Experience 9
    The Client Consultation 320
Essential Rubrics 321
Essential Review 328
*Essential Discoveries
and Accomplishments* 335

CHAPTER 20

SKIN DISEASES & DISORDERS 336

Essential Objectives 336
*Essential Histology of the Skin: Why do
I need to learn about skin diseases and
disorders when I really want to specialize
as a hair designer?* 337
*Essential Concepts: What do I need to
know about the histology of the skin in
order to perform professionally as a
cosmetologist?* 338
Essential Experience 1
    Primary and Secondary Lesions 339
Essential Experience 2
    Crossword Puzzle........................... 340
Essential Experience 3
    Crossword Puzzle........................... 341
Essential Experience 4
    Word Search Puzzle........................ 342
Essential Review 344
*Essential Discoveries
and Accomplishments* 347

CHAPTER 21

HAIR REMOVAL...............................348

Essential Objectives 348
*Essential Hair Removal: Why do I need to
learn about removing unwanted hair when
I may never provide such a service?* 349
*Essential Concepts: What do I need to
know about hair removal in order to
provide a quality service?* 350
Essential Experience 1
    Temporary and Permanent Methods
    of Hair Removal 351

Essential Experience 2
Crossword Puzzle—
Removing Unwanted Hair 352
Essential Experience 3
Matching Exercise 354
Essential Experience 4
Tweezing Eyebrows..................... 355
Essential Rubrics 357
Essential Review............................. 361
*Essential Discoveries
and Accomplishments* 363

CHAPTER 22

FACIALS.................................364
Essential Objectives........................... 364
*Essential Theory of Massage: Why do I
need to know about the underlying theory
of massage, and are facials really that
important in my career as a professional
cosmetologist?*................................. 365
*Essential Concepts: What do I need
to know about the theory of massage and
facials in order to provide quality services
to my clients?*................................. 366
Essential Experience 1
Motor Nerve Points 367
Essential Experience 2
Matching Exercise 368
Essential Experience 3
Massage Manipulations 369
Essential Experience 4
Word Scramble........................... 370
Essential Experience 5
Crossword Puzzle........................ 371
Essential Experience 6
Massage Movements 372
Essential Experience 7
Word Scramble........................... 373
Essential Experience 8
Mind Map................................. 374
Essential Experience 9
Client Consultation..................... 375
Essential Experience 10
Crossword Puzzle........................ 377

Essential Experience 11
Skin Care Product Research 378
Essential Experience 12
Facial Steaming 379
Essential Rubrics 380
Essential Review............................. 385
*Essential Discoveries
and Accomplishments* 389

CHAPTER 23

FACIAL MAKEUP 390
Essential Objectives........................... 390
*Essential Facial Makeup: What makes
applying makeup such a critical part of
my career as a cosmetologist?*............... 391
*Essential Concepts: What do I need to
know about facial makeup in order to
provide a quality service?*..................... 392
Essential Experience 1
Commercial Cosmetics.................... 393
Essential Experience 2
Windowpane—Face Shapes............. 394
Essential Experience 3
Word Scramble........................... 395
Essential Experience 4
Corrective Lip Treatment 397
Essential Experience 5
Crossword Puzzle......................... 398
Essential Experience 6
Band Lash Procedure 399
Essential Rubrics 401
Essential Review............................. 403
*Essential Discoveries
and Accomplishments* 406

CHAPTER 24

NAIL DISEASES & DISORDERS 407
Essential Objectives........................... 407
*Essential Nail Structure and Growth:
I want to be a hairstylist, not a scientist
or doctor; why do I need to learn about
nail diseases and disorders?*.................. 408

Essential Concepts: What do I need to know about nail diseases and disorders in order to provide quality manicuring and pedicuring services? 409

Essential Experience 1
Windowpane 410

Essential Experience 2
Nail Disorders, Irregularities, and Diseases 411

Essential Experience 3
Matching Exercise—Technical Terms Versus Common Terms 413

Essential Experience 4
Word Search 414

Essential Experience 5
Word Search 415

Essential Experience 6
Technical Term Mnemonics 416

Essential Review 417

Essential Discoveries and Accomplishments 419

CHAPTERS 25 & 26
MANICURING AND PEDICURING 420

Essential Objectives 420

Essential Manicuring and Pedicuring: Why are manicuring and pedicuring so important in my career as a cosmetologist? 422

Essential Concepts: What do I need to know about manicuring and pedicuring in order to provide a quality service? 423

Essential Experience 1
Windowpane—Nail Shapes 424

Essential Experience 2
Implements 425

Essential Experience 3
Matching Exercise 426

Essential Experience 4
Manicure Table Setup 427

Essential Experience 5
Word Scramble 428

Essential Experience 6
Manicure Table Setup Procedure 429

Essential Experience 7
Manicure Procedure 430

Essential Experience 8
Partners for Pedicure 431

Essential Rubrics 432

Essential Review 436

Essential Discoveries and Accomplishments 439

CHAPTERS 27 — 29
ADVANCED NAIL TECHNIQUES 440

Essential Objectives 440

Essential Advanced Nail Techniques: Why do I need to learn about advanced nail techniques to be successful? 442

Essential Concepts: What do I need to know about advanced nail techniques in order to provide a quality service? 443

Essential Experience 1
Windowpane 444

Essential Experience 2
Pre- and Post-Service Procedures 445

Essential Experience 3
Nail Tip Procedure 446

Essential Experience 4
Word Scramble 447

Essential Experience 5
Word Search 449

Essential Experience 6
Client Consultation 451

Essential Experience 7
Acrylic (Methacrylate) Nail Enhancements Using Forms 452

Essential Rubrics 455

Essential Review 459

Essential Discoveries and Accomplishments 464

CHAPTER 30
SEEKING EMPLOYMENT 465
Essential Objectives 465
Essential Employment Seeking: Why do I need to learn about seeking employment while I am still in training? 466
Essential Concepts: What do I need to know about seeking employment in order to achieve success in my career? 467
Essential Experience 1
    Personal Data Page 468
Essential Experience 2
    Mind Map—The Steps in Seeking Employment 469
Essential Experience 3
    Windowpane— Clinic Achievements 470
Essential Experience 4
    Cover Letter 471
Essential Experience 5
    Interview Preparation 472
Essential Experience 6
    Word Scramble 474
Essential Experience 7
    Why I Chose Cosmetology 475
Essential Review 476
Essential Discoveries and Accomplishments 479

CHAPTER 31
ON THE JOB 480
Essential Objectives 480
On the Job Essentials: Why do I need to learn about making the transition from school to work? 481
Essential Concepts: What do I need to know about making the transition from school to work in order to maintain satisfaction and success on the job? 482
Essential Experience 1
    Evaluate Your Skills— Are You Job Ready? 483

Essential Experience 2
    Technical Skills Improvement 485
Essential Experience 3
    Career Management 486
Essential Experience 4
    Planning Your Future 487
Essential Experience 5
    Teamwork 488
Essential Experience 6
    The Job Description 489
Essential Review 490
Essential Discoveries and Accomplishments 492

CHAPTER 32
THE SALON BUSINESS 493
Essential Objectives 493
Essential Salon Business: Is the knowledge of business really so important to someone who just wants to be a hair designer? 494
Essential Concepts: What do I need to know about the salon business in order to be successful? 495
Essential Experience 1
    Salon Research 496
Essential Experience 2
    Matching—Regulations, Business Law, and Insurance 497
Essential Experience 3
    Income and Expense 498
Essential Experience 4
    Daily Revenue Report Form 499
Essential Experience 5
    Job Descriptions 499
Essential Experience 6
    Advertising 500
Essential Experience 7
    Crossword Puzzle 501
Essential Experience 8
Interviewing Personnel 503
Essential Review 504
Essential Discoveries and Accomplishments 506

PREFACE

Introduction

Congratulations! As a student of cosmetology you now hold in your hands one of the most essential tools available to successfully progress through your course of study. You have chosen to embark upon a career in cosmetology, which can be a life-transforming event. In that journey you deserve the best possible education, which can be accomplished by using the best possible educational tools available. The *Milady's Standard Cosmetology Study Guide: The Essential Companion* is just such a tool.

PURPOSE

The purpose of the *Study Guide* is to help you, the student, to achieve the objectives of each lesson presented by your instructors. Each chapter is designed to be a critical companion to the chapter you are assigned in the *Milady's Standard Cosmetology* textbook. The study guide is designed to emphasize active, conceptual learning and to consolidate your understanding of the textbook. Information presented is provided in an informal tone, allowing the *Study Guide* to take on the role of a private tutor or companion to aid you in mastering the textbook content.

DESIGN

Each chapter of the *Study Guide* is divided into six sections as follows:

ESSENTIAL OBJECTIVES

The objectives set forth for the textbook chapter are restated to help you focus on the goals for the lesson.

ESSENTIAL SUBJECT

This section provides a brief overview about why the subject matter contained in the chapter is essential in the life of a successful cosmetologist.

ESSENTIAL CONCEPTS

This section provides an outline or brief overview of the chapter content.

ESSENTIAL EXPERIENCES

This section contains activities, projects, and puzzles that are designed to reinforce the content contained in the textbook chapter and increase your retention of the material studied. The Essential Experiences are designed to help you retain important information on a given subject through fun and interesting activities. The activities include personal research projects, mind mapping, windowpaning, matching exercises, crossword puzzles, word search puzzles, word scramble puzzles, role-playing, and so much more.

To help you understand some of the active learning exercises you will use, a brief explanation is provided here. Mind mapping is used for developing an innovative and more creative approach to thinking. It simply creates a free-flowing outline of material or information. It is easy to learn, and when you master the technique you will be able to organize an entire project or chapter in a matter of minutes. Mind mapping will allow you to release your creativity and engage both hemispheres of your brain. This technique has proved more effective than the linear form of note taking for most students. When mind mapping, the central or main idea is more clearly defined. The map lays out the relative importance of each idea or element of the subject matter. For example, the more important ideas or material will be nearer the center, and the less important material will be located in the outer parameters. Proximity and connections are used to establish the links between key concepts or ideas. The result is that review and recall will occur more quickly and be more effective. As you develop the art of mind mapping, you will see that each one takes on a unique appearance, which even adds to your recall ability of different topics or

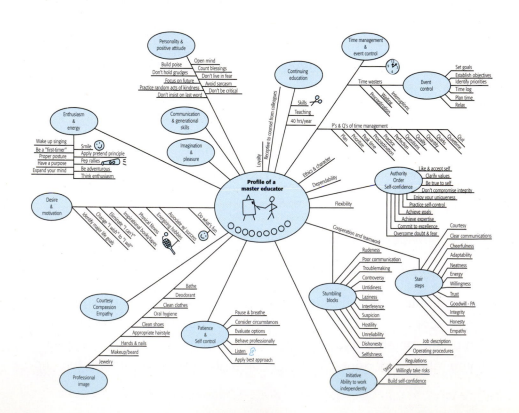

subjects. An example of how all the qualities, skills, and characteristics of an educator could be placed in a mind map is provided below.

Windowpaning is the process of transferring key elements, points, or steps in a lesson into visual images that are then hand sketched into the squares or "panes" of a matrix. Your mind thinks in pictures or images. Research indicates that people can retain in their short-term memory an average of seven bits of information with a variation of two on the plus or minus side. Therefore, it is recommended that you complete windowpanes with no more than nine panes

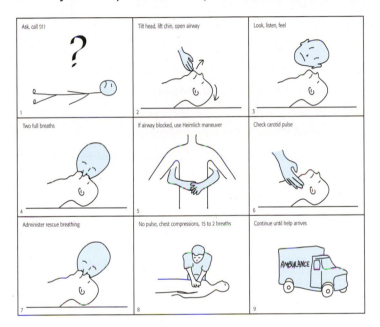

for a given topic. Refer to the example of a windowpane on how to perform cardiopulmonary resuscitation (CPR).

ESSENTIAL REVIEW

This section contains a quiz, which may include multiple choice or completion questions, designed to help you measure your understanding of the key concepts presented in the textbook chapter.

ESSENTIAL DISCOVERIES AND ACCOMPLISHMENTS

This section is simply your personal journal regarding the material studied. It is suggested that you jot notes about the concepts in the chapter that were the hardest for your to understand or remember. Next, consider yourself in the role of "teacher" and think about what you would tell your students to help them *discover* and understand those difficult concepts. It is suggested that you share your Essential Discoveries with other students in your class to determine whether what you have discovered is also beneficial to them. As a result of feedback from other students, you may want to revise your journal and include some of the good ideas received from their peers. Under Accomplishments, list at least three things you have accomplished since your last entry that relate to their career goals.

You may find it helpful to read the Essential Subject and Essential Concepts found in the *Study Guide* before reading the actual chapter in the textbook. Upon completion of the chapter, you will then want to complete the Essential Experiences, Review, and Discoveries and Accomplishments.

By choosing an institution that uses educational materials published by Milady, a part of Cengage Learning, the industry leader in cosmetology education and technology, you have taken a significant step toward a rewarding and successful career. You have chosen proven performance and longevity by choosing Milady. You have chosen wisely and well. May success and good fortune accompany you in every step you take with *Milady's Standard Cosmetology* and the *Milady's Standard Cosmetology Study Guide.* We believe that with the right tools, your commitment to the best education possible and your passion for an exciting industry, you will experience all the joys and rewards possible in a great career!

COMBINED CHAPTERS

Please note that this edition of the *Study Guide* contains information and activities related to every chapter of *Milady's Standard Cosmetology,* 2008 edition. However, for the sake of efficiency and clarity, the Manicuring and Pedicuring chapters have been combined in this *Study Guide.* In addition, the advanced nail chapters (Nail Tips, Wraps, & No-Light Gels; Acrylic [Methacrylate] Nails; and UV Gels) have also been combined.

Best wishes for success!

Letha Barnes, Director
The Career Institute
Delmar, Cengage Learning

Acknowledgments

My thanks to Lisha Barnes, my step-daughter and colleague, who has provided effort, input, ideas, and feedback for this project. Her support and loyalty are greatly appreciated.

HISTORY & CAREER OPPORTUNITIES

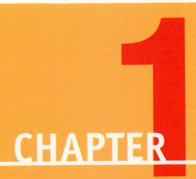

A Motivating Moment: "The person who gets the farthest is generally the one who is willing to do and dare. The sure-thing boat never gets far from shore."
—Dale Carnegie

ESSENTIAL OBJECTIVES

After studying this chapter and completing the Essential Companion components, you should be able to:

1. Describe the early origins of appearance enhancement.

2. Describe the advancements made in cosmetology during the 19th, 20th, and 21st centuries.

3. List the career opportunities available to a licensed cosmetologist.

ESSENTIAL HISTORY AND OPPORTUNITIES

Why is knowing about this history and evolution of this industry so important to my success in cosmetology or a related field?

As a professional in this industry, your overall knowledge about the field in general will impact your credibility with your clients and help you serve them better. A study of the trends throughout history will also establish that many repeat themselves, either decades or centuries later. Thus, the more you know about the history of cosmetology, the more prepared you will be for the changing trends throughout your career.

Society as a whole now has access to professional hair, skin, and nail care services. Therefore, it is important for today's professional to also know about all the various career paths available to you in order to determine which one best suits you.

What are the essentials about the industry's history and the career opportunities available?

Nearly every society has found it necessary to confine, cut, or manage the hair in order to keep it out of the way. The human species has essentially always had a basic desire to look good. As we look at history, that desire for personal adornment has varied in form from the ornately curled, blond wigs of Roman matrons to the sleek, waved heads of the flappers in the 1920s.

In pre-industrial societies, hairstyling was used to indicate a person's social status. For example, primitive men would fasten bones, feathers, and other items into their hair for the purpose of impressing the lowly and frightening the enemy with their rank and prowess. Caesar made the noblemen of ancient Gaul cut off their hair as a sign of submission after he conquered them. In addition, occupational associations have been indicated by hair over history as manifested by the gray wigs worn by the barristers of England and the lacquered, black wigs worn by Japanese geisha.

Hair arrangement has also been used to indicate age or marital status. Adolescence was shown by shaved heads for young Hindu men, while boys in ancient Greece simply cut their hair. Until the 20th century, generally only the upper classes enjoyed fashionable hairstyles. However, in the first half of the 20th century, nearly all classes of women followed the trend set by film stars like Jean Harlow or Marilyn Monroe.

Because of the general increase in wealth, the improvement of mass communication, greater individualism, and overall attitude of informality, men and women of all classes can choose the style and color of hair that suits their interests, their needs, and their best image. This change in perspective has greatly increased the demand for the services of licensed professionals in the cosmetology industry.

Historical Time Line

Using the material contained in the textbook and any other resources available to you to create a visual time line of the history of hairdressing from the beginning of recorded history to the present. The top of the line will indicate the year, decade, or century and the bottom of the time line will contain drawings or pictures (cut and pasted) of hairstyles or tools and implements that represent that era.

Use large poster board, colored markers, and any other items you can think of to re-create the history of hairdressing in a colorful and interesting manner. Additional historical data is provided here.

The Ice Age	Haircutting and styling were practiced; implements were shaped from sharpened flints, oyster shells, or bone; animal strips of hide were used to tie hair back or as adornment.
4000 BC	Ancient Egyptians used cosmetics for personal beautification, religious ceremonies, and burial ceremonies.
1500 BC	Henna, a dye extracted from the leaves of an ornamental shrub, was used extensively to impart a reddish hue to the hair and nails.
300 BC	Hairstyling was introduced in Rome; women used hair color to indicate class: noblewomen tinted their hair red, middle-class colored their hair blond, and poor women colored their hair black.
Renaissance	(Began in the 14th century and lasted into the 17th century.) Particular emphasis was placed on physical appearance. Hair was carefully dressed and ornaments and headdresses were worn.
1450	Barbering and surgery were separated by law.
1541	Henry VIII reunited barbers and surgeons of London by granting a charter to the Company of Barber Surgeons.

1

ESSENTIAL EXPERIENCE *continued*

1892	Frenchman Alexandre F. Godefroy invented the hot-blast hair dryer.
1905	Charles Nessler invented the first electric perm machine.
1906	Sarah Breedlove married C. J. Walker, who began selling her scalp conditioning and healing treatment called "Madam Walker's Wonderful Hair Grower."
1910	Madam C. J. Walker moved her company to Indianapolis where she built a factory, a hair salon, and a training school.
1932	Ralph L. Evans and Everett G. McDonough pioneered a perm method using external heat generated by a chemical reaction.
1941	Scientists developed the "cold wave" method of perming hair.
Today	Hair color, texture, and style prevail.

2

ESSENTIAL EXPERIENCE

Mind Mapping

Mind mapping simply creates a free-flowing outline of material or information with the central or key point being located in the center. (Refer to the Preface for more details on how to create a mind map.) The key point of this mind map is you as a licensed cosmetologist. Diagram the different career opportunities awaiting you upon your completion of the cosmetology course. Identify the different disciplines and branches of each, including the different positions that may be obtained in that field. Use terms, pictures, and symbols as desired. Using color will increase the mind's retention and memory of the information. Keep your mind open and uncluttered and don't worry about where a line or word should go. The organization of the map will usually take care of itself.

3 ESSENTIAL EXPERIENCE

Character Study and Report

Select a 20th-century industry icon (such as Vidal Sassoon, John Paul DeJoria, or Robert Cromeans) and conduct research on their life and career in cosmetology. Again, use the library, the Internet, trade magazines, or other resources to obtain your information. Explain the impact this person has had on the industry and why or why not he/she should be respected within the industry. Don't limit yourself to a written report. Feel free to use illustrations, photos, drawings, diagrams, and color to enhance your report and make it more meaningful.

ESSENTIAL EXPERIENCE

Word Scramble

Using the clues provided, unscramble the terms below.

Scramble	Correct Word
msiekksoto	_ _ _ _ _ _ _ _ _ _
	Clue: Greek term.
mngipste	_ _ _ _ _ _ _ _
	Clue: Made from berries.
tsreyo lesshl	_ _ _ _ _ _ _ _ _ _ _ _
	Clue: Used to make implements.
mlaain wsine	_ _ _ _ _ _ _ _ _ _ _
	Clue: Used to tie hair back.
feemprsu	_ _ _ _ _ _ _ _
	Clue: Used in Grecian religious rites.
nniarcba	_ _ _ _ _ _ _ _
	Clue: Made into red pigment.
laemtoa	_ _ _ _ _ _ _
	Clue: Used to make masks.
zttdrusiiiaaonniusl	_ _ _ _ _ _ _ _ _ _ _ _ _ _ _ _ _ _ _
	Clue: Brought new prosperity.
aapetrclo	_ _ _ _ _ _ _ _ _
	Clue: Stained nails warm red.
selarhc noserv	_ _ _ _ _ _ _ _ _ _ _ _ _
	Clue: Formulated nail lacquer.

ESSENTIAL REVIEW

Using the following words, fill in the blanks below to form a thorough review of Chapter 1: Cosmetology. Words or terms may be used more than once or not at all.

austere	dentistry	kohl	spa
barber	desire	lacquered	stone
bare brow	educators	leaves	surgery
beeswax	esthetician	lips	texture
berries	fastest-growing	nuts	towering
black	fourteenth	pancake	headdresses
bloodletting	full-service salon	processes	tree bark
braiding	hair color	pulling teeth	trends
classes	ice	red	
curl	irons	restrictive	

ESSENTIAL REVIEW *continued*

1. If business is your calling, you will find that management opportunities in the salon and _____ environment are quite diverse.

2. Archeological studies reveal that haircutting and hairstyling were practiced in some form as early as the _____ age.

3. Ancient records show that coloring matter was made from minerals, insects, _____ , herbs, and leaves to color the hair, skin, and nails.

4. Roman noblewomen tinted their hair _____ .

5. During the golden age of Greece, women applied white lead on their faces, _____ on their eyes, and vermillion on their cheeks and lips.

6. The poor class of ancient Rome wore their hair _____ .

7. The modern barber pole was originally the symbol of the _____ surgeon.

8. Up until the 19th century, _____ was performed by barbers.

9. The barber pole has its roots in the medical procedure known as _____ .

10. The Middle Ages showed women wearing _____ .

11. During the Renaissance, a _____ was thought to give women a look of greater intelligence.

12. The Victorian Age was one of the most austere and _____ periods in history.

13. Nail color was popular in China in 3000 BC when aristocrats rubbed a tinted mixture of gum Arabic, gelatin, _____ , and egg whites onto their nails to turn them crimson or ebony.

14. In 1935, Max Factor created _____ makeup to make actors' skin look natural on color film.

15. Beyond defining your area of expertise, you must also decide whether or not you want to work in a specialty salon, _____ , or day spa.

ESSENTIAL DISCOVERIES AND ACCOMPLISHMENTS

In the space below, jot some notes about what concepts of this chapter were hardest for you to understand or remember. Imagine finding yourself suddenly in the role of "teacher" and consider what you would tell your "students" about these concepts. Share your Essential Discoveries with some of the other students in your class and ask if they are helpful to them. You may want to revise your discoveries based on any good ideas shared by your peers.

Discoveries:

_____

_____

_____

_____

_____

_____

_____

_____

_____

List at least three things you have accomplished since you to decided to enroll in school.

Accomplishments:

_____

_____

_____

_____

LIFE SKILLS

CHAPTER **2**

A Motivating Moment: "The greatest discovery of any generation is that a human being can alter his life by altering his attitude."—William James

ESSENTIAL OBJECTIVES

After studying this chapter and completing the Essential Companion components, you should be able to:

1. List the principles that contribute to personal and professional success.

2. Explain the concept of self-management.

3. Create a personal mission statement.

4. Explain how to set long- and short-term goals.

5. Discuss the most effective ways to manage time.

6. Describe good study habits.

7. Define *ethics.*

8. List the characteristics of a healthy, positive attitude.

ESSENTIAL LIFE SKILLS

Why do I need to learn about life skills in order to be successful as a cosmetologist?

Life skills are essential for increasing your effectiveness, career success, and personal satisfaction in your personal life as well as on the job. You may be able to achieve the highest quality technical skills, but if you are unable to manage the "big picture" of your life in general, those technical skills will be yield little or no results.

For example, research shows that stress has reached epidemic proportions in the United States and is having a negative impact on all of society, especially in the workplace, even in the field of cosmetology. Our goal in this chapter is to provide ideas, tools, and the best practices that you can use to increase your effectiveness, enhance your career, and feel more fulfilled with your life in general.

ESSENTIAL CONCEPTS OF LIFE SKILLS MANAGEMENT

What do I need to know about life skills management in order to be effective as a licensed professional?

Managing your life skills includes a plethora of qualities, characteristics, and skills. In addition to all the technical skills you will need to master for your new career, you will need to practice general principles that form the foundation for both personal and business success. You will need to understand personal motivation and what is meant by self-management.

You will develop skills useful in expanding your creativity. Yale psychologist Robert Sternberg argues that successful intelligence goes beyond cognitive intelligence to include what he calls creative and practical intelligence. He says that people with creative intelligence know how to leverage their cognitive intelligence by *applying* what they learn in *new* and *creative* ways. Therefore, this chapter introduces you to some strategies that will help you do just that. Goal setting is an integral part of any successful person's career. Thus, you need to learn how to set goals, monitor them, and expand them throughout your journey.

All of these life skills will be better managed if you also learn how to manage the events in your life. By event control, we really mean what has long been referred to as time management. Tips from the experts on time management will be useful in planning your personal quest for success.

You are now enrolled in a career program of study. Therefore, you will need to ensure that your personal study skills are up-to-speed and adequate to see you successfully through the course. You will even need to identify your own personal learning style in order to maximize the time spent in both study and in the classroom.

You will realize after completion of this chapter that other key ingredients to success are affected by your personality, your attitude, your approach to professional ethics, and, possibly more than anything else, your ability to interact effectively with others, which is also known as human relations. Your future will be much richer if you look at your training as the opportunity to learn to manage your life in the same manner as those successful professionals who have attained many of the goals you aspire to achieve.

1

Goals Setting

If you have not already done so, make a chart of your short- and long-term goals as well as your action plan for achievement of those goals in the space provided. Your action plan should include the education you need to attain as well as target dates for completion. Remember a goal is anything you can *have, be,* or *do.* For most people, goals are divided into several categories, including: Career/Job, Salary/Earnings, Personal/Family Relationship, Health/Weight, Education/Skills, Knowledge, Free-Personal Time, Travel, Financial/Material Assets, Home, Transportation, Spirituality. (Make you own chart if more space is needed.)

Short-Term Goals: Less Than 1 Year	Long-Term Goals: 1 to 10 Years	Action Plan: Education Required

2

2
ESSENTIAL EXPERIENCE

Collage of Goals

It is a well-known belief that in order to obtain goals, we need to visualize ourselves as having already attained them. Therefore, we should picture ourselves at that desired weight, or driving that fancy sports car that appeals to us, or living in that special home we want. With that in mind, and referring back to the goals you set for yourself in Essential Experience 1, create a collage that depicts having attained that success. For example, if you have a special home in mind, cut out a picture that represents that dream and paste it on a poster board. If you have a goal of driving a Jaguar, find a picture of a Jaguar in a magazine and cut it out and park it in front of the house. Cut out a picture of yourself as well and place it in the Jag!

If you dream of having a wonderful spouse and two children, cut out a picture of that "significant other" and two children and yourself and place them in front of the house as well. Perhaps you will have a picture of a successful platform artist performing on stage with your head overlaid on the body! Get the idea? Once you have completed the collage that holds all your dreams and goals, place it in a prominent place in your life where you will see it each and every day. By seeing yourself in those circumstances, your subconscious works even harder to help you accomplish the activities set out in your action plan and finally reach your goals.

3

Mind Map of Yourself Today

Mind mapping simply creates a free-flowing outline of material or information with the central or key point being located in the center. (Refer to the Preface for more details on how to create a mind map.) The key point of this mind map is you, as a student. Diagram the different aspects of your life as they exist today. Use terms, pictures, and symbols as desired. Using color will increase your mind's retention and memory of the information. Keep your mind open and uncluttered and don't worry about where a line or word should go. The organization of the map will usually take care of itself.

For example, draw a picture of yourself in a circle in the middle of the page. Draw a line out from the center and insert another circle where you write "student." Off the student circle, you will draw lines that might say things like attend class, study, work with clients, etc. Another line from the center circle might say Mom or Dad (if you are a parent), and the lines off that circle might reflect your role as a parent with tasks like drive car pool, coach little league, etc. Consider all the aspects of your life and put them into the mind map in the space provided.

ESSENTIAL EXPERIENCE

Mind Map Your Future

Using the collage you created in Essential Experience 2, create another mind map using the guidelines presented in the previous exercise. This time, however, draw the map as you see yourself in 10 years. Upon completion of these drawings, place them in a safe place for reflection later. You may want to take another look at the end of your course of study and then on New Year's Day each year until the time that you had scheduled for reaching those goals you defined in Essential Experience 1.

5

Track Your Attendance

Managing your life skills also includes something called "impulse management." In this context, impulses are defined as anything that isn't an integral part of your goals and may actually interfere with the accomplishment of your goals. According to *Webster's,* a goal is defined as "an end that one strives to attain." An impulse is defined as a "sudden inclination to act." History indicates that students often act on impulse when they decide to not attend school as scheduled. With that in mind, consider tracking your attendance one month at a time using the following form. This will give you clear, first-hand documentation if your are committed to achieving your goals or you are letting "impulse management" rule your life.

Date	Hours Missed	Reason for Absence	If action was "impulse management," what actions will prevent the absence in the future?

6

Self-Assessment of Personal Characteristics

Consider the qualities and characteristics you now possess and list them either as strengths or weaknesses in the space provided. If the characteristic is a strength, state the benefits received from it. If the characteristic is a weakness, identify steps you can take to improve. Refer to the example to get started.

Strength	Benefit	Weakness	Action Plan
Promptness	Maximum use of my time; respect from others.	Tardiness	Get up earlier; implement better time-management strategies; be more conscientious and respectful of those who are expecting me on time.

7 ESSENTIAL EXPERIENCE

Time Management

For one week, track your time in 30 minute increments. While this may seem like a drudgery and cause you to groan, you will find the results totally enlightening. Take a look at how much time you spent in class, how much time you spent (or didn't spend) studying, how much time you spent eating and sleeping, how much quality time you spent with your family, and how much time you lost on unimportant activities, etc.

Time Utilization Log

Time	Sun	Mon	Tue	Wed	Thu	Fri	Sat
7:00 am							
7:30 am							
8:00 am							
8:30 am							
9:00 am							
9:30 am							
10:00 am							
10:30 am							
11:00 am							
11:30 am							
12:00 pm							
12:30 pm							
1:00 pm							
1:30 pm							
2:00 pm							
2:30 pm							
3:00 pm							
3:30 pm							
4:00 pm							

7

ESSENTIAL EXPERIENCE *continued*

Time Utilization Log						
4:30 pm						
5:00 pm						
5:30 pm						
6:00 pm						
6:30 pm						
7:00 pm						
7:30 pm						
8:00 pm						
8:30 pm						
9:00 pm						
9:30 pm						
10:00 pm						
10:30 pm						
11:00 pm						

8

Action Plan for Time Management

After you have analyzed the time utilization log thoroughly, develop a personal action plan (using the chart below) for better managing your time in the following week. To help you do that, you need to identify the activities you wish to complete in the next seven days. Then you need to prioritize those activities as A—greatest importance; B—average importance; C—least importance. As you progress through the week, indicate when each of the tasks has been completed.

Priorities for the Current Week		
Activities to Complete	Priority Rank	Date Completed

9
ESSENTIAL EXPERIENCE

Is Your Bad Attitude an Addiction?

Experts tell us that the first step in addressing any addiction is recognizing, defining, and admitting the problem. Definitions: **Addict**—to devote or surrender (oneself) to something habitually or obsessively. **Addiction**—the compulsive need for (or dependence on) and use of a habit-forming substance (or behavior) characterized by tolerance and by well-defined physiological symptoms upon withdrawal. **Dependence**—the quality or state of being subordinate to something else. Please answer the following questions as honestly as you can.

1. Do you lose productive time due to your bad attitude?   ___ **Yes** ___ **No**

2. Is your bad attitude making your home life unhappy?   ___ **Yes** ___ **No**

3. Have you ever felt remorse because of your bad attitude?   ___ **Yes** ___ **No**

4. Have you gotten into financial difficulties because of your bad attitude?   ___ **Yes** ___ **No**

5. Do you turn to lower companions and an inferior environment because of your bad attitude?   ___ **Yes** ___ **No**

6. Does your bad attitude make you careless with your family's welfare.   ___ **Yes** ___ **No**

7. Has your ambition decreased because of your bad attitude?   ___ **Yes** ___ **No**

8. Does your bad attitude cause you difficulty in sleeping?   ___ **Yes** ___ **No**

9. Has your efficiency ever decreased because of your bad attitude?   ___ **Yes** ___ **No**

10. Is your bad attitude jeopardizing your job or business?   ___ **Yes** ___ **No**

9
ESSENTIAL EXPERIENCE *continued*

11. Do you use your bad attitude to escape from worries
    or troubles? ___ **Yes** ___ **No**

12. Have you ever experienced memory loss due to your
    bad attitude? ___ **Yes** ___ **No**

13. Has your supervisor ever counseled you because of your
    bad attitude? ___ **Yes** ___ **No**

14. Is your bad attitude an absolute must in your daily life? ___ **Yes** ___ **No**

15. Have you ever been to a hospital or institution because
    of your bad attitude? ___ **Yes** ___ **No**

If you have answered yes to any ONE of these questions, this is a definite
warning that you may be dependent upon your bad attitude.

If you answered yes to any TWO of these questions, the chances that you are
dependent on your bad attitude are high.

If you answered yes to THREE or more, you definitely are dependent upon
your bad attitude.

To begin immediate recovery from this dependency, *smile,* think positive
thoughts, speak positive self-affirmations, and visualize personal health,
happiness, and success!

Questions adapted from Johns Hopkins University Hospital.

ESSENTIAL REVIEW

Using the following words, fill in the blanks below to form a thorough review of Chapter 2: Life Skills. Words or terms may be used more than once or not at all.

accomplishment	down time	personality	strengths
attitude	education	prioritized	technical
caring	energetic	problem-solving	test
communication	game plan	procrastination	time-out
competent	integrity	professional	uninterrupted
creative	long-term	respect	values
desire	moral	self-esteem	visualize
discipline	motivation	short-term	vocabulary
discretion	passion	small tasks	
diplomacy	perfectionism	social	

1. By nature, the salon is a _____ workplace where you are expected to exercise your artistic talent.

2. One important life skill is that of being genuinely _____ and helpful to other people.

3. Another necessary life skill is that of maintaining a cooperative _____ in all situations.

4. You can have all the talent in the world and still not be successful if your talent is not fueled by the _____ for your work that will sustain you over the course of your career.

5. _____ is based on inner strength and begins with trusting your ability to reach your goals.

6. The more you _____ yourself as a success, the easier it is to turn your goals into realities.

7. Principles or guidelines for helping you achieve success include building on your _____ , being kind to yourself, defining success as you see it, practicing new behaviors, and separating your personal life from your work.

8. Successful people make a point of relating to everyone they know with a conscious feeling of _____ .

9. _____ keeps you from maintaining peak performance.

ESSENTIAL REVIEW *continued*

10. An unhealthy compulsion to do things perfectly is called
    _____ .

11. Having a _____ is the conscious act of planning your life.

12. To enhance skill creativity, you should stop criticizing yourself, stop asking
    others what to do, change your _____ , and not try to go it
    totally alone.

13. A personal mission statement sets forth the _____ you plan to
    live by and establishes future goals.

14. Goals which take several years to accomplish are called
    _____ goals.

15. To manage time more effectively, tasks should be _____ ,
    which means making a list of tasks that need to be done in the order of
    most to least important.

16. Give yourself some _____ whenever you are frustrated,
    overwhelmed, irritated, worried, or feeling guilty about something.

17. Learn _____ techniques that will save you time and needless
    frustration.

18. If you find studying overwhelming, focus on _____ .

19. Studying should take place in a quiet spot where you can study
    _____ .

20. Studying is best done when you feel _____ and motivated.

21. Retention of important material is best accomplished when you
    _____ yourself on each section of a chapter.

22. Ethics are the _____ principles of good character, proper
    conduct, and judgment we live by.

23. Self-care, integrity, and _____ and communication are key
    qualities of ethics.

24. Maintain your _____ by making sure your behavior and
    actions match your values.

25. Ingredients for a healthy, well-developed attitude include _____ ,
    soft tone of voice, emotional stability, sensitivity, high values and goals,
    receptivity, and communication skills.

ESSENTIAL DISCOVERIES AND ACCOMPLISHMENTS

In the space below, jot some notes about what concepts of this chapter were hardest for you to understand or remember. Imagine finding yourself suddenly in the role of "teacher" and consider what you would tell your "students" about these difficult concepts. Share your Essential Discoveries with some of the other students in your class and ask if they are helpful to them. You may want to revise your notes based on good ideas shared by your peers. Under Accomplishments, list at least three things you have accomplished since your last entry that relate to your career goals.

Discoveries:

_____

_____

_____

_____

_____

_____

_____

_____

_____

_____

Accomplishments:

_____

_____

_____

_____

_____

YOUR PROFESSIONAL IMAGE

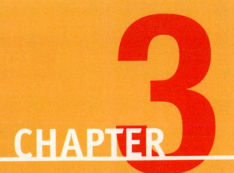

A Motivating Moment: "To simplify, you have to clarify. Simplification is the new competitive advantage."—Jack Trout

ESSENTIAL OBJECTIVES

After studying this chapter and completing the Essential Companion components, you should be able to:

1. Understand personal hygiene.

2. Explain the concept of dressing for success.

3. Use appropriate methods to ensure personal health and well-being.

4. Demonstrate an understanding of ergonomic principles and ergonomically correct postures and movements.

ESSENTIAL PROFESSIONALISM

Why are professionalism and my image so important to my success in cosmetology or a related field?

Professionalism has been defined as the conduct, aims, or qualities that characterize or mark a professional person. The cosmetology industry and all related fields such as nail technology, barbering, esthetics, and massage therapy represent the "image" industry. There is no other profession in which image and communications skills (which we will learn more about in Chapter 4) are more essential. As a student in training and as a professional you will come in contact with numerous clients on a daily basis.

Psychologists tell us that people form an opinion of us in the first few seconds of meeting us. It is up to us to make that first impression a positive one. It is also up to us to make that positive impression a lasting one. We can accomplish that by understanding how to enjoy both personal and professional health. This chapter will help you do just that.

What are the essentials about image and professional development?

As a professional licensee in the cosmetology industry or related career path, it will be essential for you to concentrate on your personal and professional health. You will need to be aware of your physical presence, your nutrition, and your ability to manage personal stress. In the process, you will realize the importance of developing a positive winning attitude and practicing professionalism at all times. Chapter 3 of the textbook and this Essential Companion will provide the road map for helping you achieve all these important personal and professional goals.

3

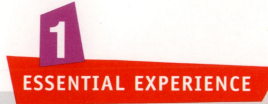

ESSENTIAL EXPERIENCE

What Does Your Professional Image Say About You?

Professional image is the impression you project and consists of your outward appearance as well as the conduct you exhibit in the workplace. It is essentially the code of behavior by which you conduct yourself. It relates to proper conduct and business dealings with employers, clients and coworkers, and others with whom you come in contact. Professionalism will help you establish a well-respected reputation. Ask yourself the following questions to help you evaluate your professionalism and your professional image.

1. Do you treat others honestly and fairly at all times?

2. Are you courteous and do you show respect for the feelings, beliefs, and rights of others?

3. Do you keep your word when you make a promise?

4. Do you set an example of good conduct and behavior at all times?

5. Are you loyal to your family, your friends, your school, and fellow students?

6. Do you obey all the rules and standards of conduct set forth by your institution?

If you answered "no" to any of the above questions, you may want to re-evaluate your commitment to a professional career. If you answered "yes" to all, give yourself a pat on the back. You practice many qualities required for projecting a professional image.

2

ESSENTIAL EXPERIENCE

Policy Development

Imagine yourself the owner of a professional establishment and write a detailed dress code that you would require all employees to follow.

Dress Code: _____

_____

_____

_____

_____

_____

_____

_____

_____

_____

_____

_____

_____

_____

_____

_____

3
ESSENTIAL EXPERIENCE

Word Scramble—Your Professional Image

Scramble	Correct Word
csexeeir	_ _ _ _ _ _ _ _
	Clue: Promotes proper functions of organs.
ggnmoior	_ _ _ _ _ _ _ _
	Clue: An extension of pesonal hygiene.
loanitaxre	_ _ _ _ _ _ _ _ _ _
	Clue: Getting away from it all.
oeptrus	_ _ _ _ _ _ _
	Clue: Position or bearing of the body.
stre	_ _ _ _
	Clue: Recovery from fatigue.
csimongreo	_ _ _ _ _ _ _ _ _ _
	Clue: The study of human characteristics for the specific work environment.
niosfesorpliamsi	_ _ _ _ _ _ _ _ _ _ _ _ _ _ _ _
	Clue: Business conduct.
ehhtal	_ _ _ _ _ _
	Clue: Well-being.
neegyih	_ _ _ _ _ _ _
	Clue: Practicing cleanliness.
ressst	_ _ _ _ _ _
	Clue: Inability to cope.
zssaceeoric	_ _ _ _ _ _ _ _ _ _ _
	Clue: Of secondary importance.

4

ESSENTIAL EXPERIENCE

Rate Your Image

On a scale of 1 to 5, with 5 considered being the best, rate your appearance in the following categories:

_____ Clothing is clean, pressed, and free of stains or damage.

_____ Dress is in compliance with the dress code established by the institution.

_____ Shoes are clean, polished, and in good repair.

_____ Makeup (if applicable) is tasteful and neatly applied.

_____ Hair is properly groomed and styled appropriately for current trends.

_____ Facial hair (beard or mustache, if applicable) is properly trimmed and neat.

_____ Hands and nails are properly manicured; nails are clean and trimmed appropriately.

_____ Fragrance is appropriate, not overpowering.

_____ Hygiene is maintained (daily bath, proper use of deodorant, teeth are brushed, etc.).

_____ Jewelry is kept to a minimum and not overdone or too trendy.

Add your scores and evaluate your image according to the following guidelines.

45–50	Your image is excellent.
40–44	Your image is above average.
30–39	Your image is average.
Below 30	Improvement is needed. Evaluate the chart and pay particular attention to any category rated less than 3. Make a personal commitment to improvement in those areas.

5

Analyze Your Personal Lifestyle

Answer the following questions thoughtfully and honestly.

1. How many hours of sleep do you get on average nightly?

2. Describe the exercise you get daily/weekly, if any.

3. What methods do you use for relaxation, and how often?

4. Describe your daily personal hygiene and grooming regimen, including the care of your hands and feet.

5. Think back over the past three days and report on your nutrition habits. What did you eat for breakfast, lunch, and dinner over that period of time?

6. Evaluate and list other lifestyle components such as the use of alcohol, tobacco, or drugs. Do they have a negative impact on your life?

As a result of the analysis of your personal lifestyle, write a Plan of Action for improving your lifestyle and habits to make the most of a healthy and balanced life, physically, mentally, and emotionally.

PLAN OF ACTION

_____

_____

_____

_____

6 ESSENTIAL EXPERIENCE

Your Attitude—What Does It Say About You?

One way to determine whether or not you possess and convey a positive attitude is to ask yourself the following questions daily. They have been adapted from a well-known poem "I Promise Myself" by an unknown author.

1. Do you promise yourself to be so strong that nothing can disturb your peace of mind?

2. Do you promise yourself to talk health, happiness, and prosperity to every person you meet?

3. Do you promise yourself to make all your friends feel that there is something special in them?

4. Do you promise yourself to look at the sunny side of everything and make your optimism come true?

5. Do you promise yourself to think only of the *best,* to work only for the *best,* and to expect only the *best?*

6. Do you promise yourself to be just as enthusiastic about the success of others as you are about your own success?

7. Do you promise yourself to forget the mistakes of the past and press on to the greater achievements of the future?

8. Do you promise yourself to wear a cheerful countenance at all times and greet every living creature you meet with a smile?

9. Do you promise yourself to give so much time to the improvement of yourself that you have no time to criticize others?

10. Do you promise yourself to be too large for worry, too noble for anger, too strong for fear, and too happy to permit the presence of trouble in your life?

If you make these ten promises daily, you will live a life full of prosperity and rewards too great to count!

ESSENTIAL REVIEW

Using the following words, fill in the blanks below to form a thorough review of Chapter 3: Your Professional Image.

balance	health	personal	stress
blend	hygiene pack	pressure	tension
callused	image	professional	thirty
disconnect	impression	repetitive	varicose veins
energy	jingle	shock absorption	work habits
ergonomics	mask	sleep	

1. Your professional image is the _____ you project and consists of your outward appearance and the conduct you exhibit in the workplace.

2. A good way to ensure that you always smell fresh and clean is to create a _____ .

3. The daily maintenance of cleanliness and healthfulness is known as _____ hygiene.

4. Stressful _____ motions have a cumulative effect on muscles and joints.

5. Physical presentation, which includes your posture, your walk, and your movements, is part of your _____ image.

6. When you obtain employment, strive to have your hair, makeup, and clothing style be consistent with the _____ of the salon.

7. Accessories are best kept simple and attractive, and jewelry should not _____ while working.

8. Makeup should accentuate your best features and _____ your less flattering ones.

9. _____ is the study of how a workplace can best be designed for comfort, safety, efficiency, and productivity.

10. An awareness of your body posture and movements, coupled with better work habits and proper tools and equipment will enhance your _____ and comfort.

ESSENTIAL DISCOVERIES AND ACCOMPLISHMENTS

In the space below, jot some notes about what concepts of this chapter were hardest for you to understand or remember. Imagine finding yourself suddenly in the role of "teacher" and consider what you would tell your "students" about these difficult concepts. Share your Essential Discoveries with some of the other students in your class and ask if they are helpful to them. You may want to revise your notes based on good ideas shared by your peers. Under Accomplishments, list at least three things you have accomplished since your last entry that relate to your career goals.

Discoveries:

_____

_____

_____

_____

_____

_____

_____

_____

_____

_____

_____

Accomplishments:

_____

_____

_____

_____

_____

COMMUNICATING FOR SUCCESS

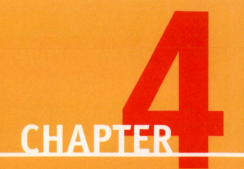

CHAPTER **4**

A Motivating Moment: "To live our lives fully, to work whole heartedly, to refuse directly what we can't swallow, to accept the mystery in all matters of meaning . . . this is the ultimate adventure."—Peter Block

ESSENTIAL OBJECTIVES

After studying this chapter and completing the Essential Companion components, you should be able to:

1. List the golden rules of human relations.

2. Explain the basic processes of effective communication.

3. Conduct a successful client consultation.

4. Handle delicate communication with your clients.

5. Build open lines of communication with coworkers and salon managers.

Why do I need to learn about communicating when I just want to cut hair?

Today's professionals, regardless of their chosen field, thrive on the exchange of information. In fact, it is information that acts as the fuel that keeps businesses going, moving, and growing. You must think of managing your career as a professional in the beauty industry as that of managing your own business. Indeed, when you build and retain a loyal clientele, you are building a successful business. Therefore, you need to receive information in order to make decisions, develop strategies, and effectively interact with your clients. You need to send information if you want your decisions and strategies to be followed and accepted.

This exchange of information is called communication. Your technical skills, however outstanding they may be, will not bring back a client who does not feel comfortable, appreciated, and important as a result of a visit to your salon. Thus, you must be able to address those important social and emotional needs through effective communications. In addition, you cannot provide those exceptional technical services if you do not truly understand the client's desires. Therefore, communication skills play a huge role in your quest for success.

What do I need to know about communicating for success in order to provide quality service to my clients and enjoy career success?

We communicate by not only speaking, but by listening as well as reading and writing. In order to exchange information with our clients about their hair, skin, and nail care needs, we must be able to exchange information effectively. We send information by speaking and writing. We receive information by listening and reading. In addition to those methods, we communicate without using words. We can send and receive messages by using gestures, facial expressions, voice changes, eye contact, personal mannerisms, dress, and posture. Throughout this whole communicating process, we are involved in relationship building. We will build relationships with our clients, with our coworkers, and with our supervisors and salon managers or owners.

Therefore, we must develop exceptional skills in conducting consultations with our clients that will result in their desired outcomes. We must learn to interact effectively on a day-to-day basis with our peers and coworkers in order to participate in a highly productive, team-oriented environment. And, finally, we must know how to respond to and interact favorably with our supervisors in order to ensure our continued career development and growth.

1

ESSENTIAL EXPERIENCE

Body Language Matching Exercise

Every part of our body has something to add to the message we are trying to send. Hand movements are the most common companions to spoken messages, more so for some than others. Many hand movements are so common they have come to mean the same thing for all of us. From the list below, match the listed hand movements with the nonverbal message they send.

1. Pointing a finger at someone.   ____ Boredom, nervousness

2. Twiddling thumbs.   ____ A warning, an accusation

3. Clasping two hands overhead.   ____ Hopefulness

4. Drumming or tapping fingers.   ____ Calmness, self-confidence

5. Crossing two fingers.   ____ A threat

6. Crossing arms across chest.   ____ Impatience, annoyance

7. Folding hands together on desk.   ____ "Okay" or "right on"

8. Making a circle with thumb   ____ Authority, anger
                                                          and forefinger.

9. Making a fist.   ____ Victory

4

2

Eye Movement

As with our hands, we can use our eyes to send nonverbal messages which might include close attention, anger, admiration, disbelief or surprise. Study the list of various eye movements below and write in the space provided the nonverbal message you believe the eye movement sends.

Staring and having a tightened jaw _____

Rolling the eyes _____

Looking directly at someone _____

Opening the eyes wide _____

Staring/glaring at someone for too long _____

Blinking eyes rapidly _____

Looking directly at strangers in close quarters _____

Shifting eyes away to avoid direct contact _____

4

Mind Map Consultation Interference

Mind mapping simply creates a free-flowing outline of material or information with the central or key point being located in the center. The key point of this mind map is a client consultation. Diagram all the things that could interfere with the communication process during a client consultation. Use terms, pictures, and symbols as desired. Use color to increase the mind's retention and memory of the material. Keep your mind open and uncluttered and don't worry about where a line or word should go as the organization of the map will usually take care of itself.

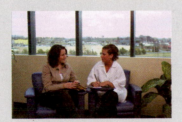

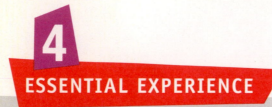

4 ESSENTIAL EXPERIENCE

Partner Messaging

Choose another student as your partner and conduct this communication exercise. Spend 5 minutes talking to each other about any subject you choose. Interact openly and respond to each other naturally. At the conclusion of the 5 minutes, each of you should make a list of the messages you received. Then review the lists together and compare the messages received to the messages you each intended to send. List the results in the space provided.

Message Received	Message Intended
_____	_____
_____	_____
_____	_____
_____	_____
_____	_____
_____	_____
_____	_____
_____	_____

5

ESSENTIAL EXPERIENCE

Role Playing a Dissatisfied Client

The purpose of role playing is to help you understand the views and feelings of other people with respect to a wide range of personal and social issues. By acting out situations in which people are in conflict, you can begin to understand the other person's point of view. In this activity, there will be three main characters and several other students will be needed to observe. Three of you will perform the role playing exercise while the other students observe and make notes. Upon completion of the role play, ask the observers what they saw, what worked in the communication exchange, what did not work, and why.

One student will role play the salon stylist, another student will play a client who has come into the salon for a haircolor service and is clearly dissatisfied with the results. The third character will be the salon supervisor who ultimately has to become involved in the quest for a solution. Upon completion of the role play and discussion with the observers, record your findings from the activity in the space provided. Consider answering the following questions: What did you learn from this experience? Are there certain ways to handle conflict that are more effective than others? If so, what are they and why do they work better?

_____

_____

_____

_____

_____

_____

_____

_____

_____

_____

_____

6

ESSENTIAL EXPERIENCE

Windowpane—Client Consultation Tools

Windowpaning is the process of transferring key elements, points, or steps in a lesson into visual images that are hand sketched into the squares or "panes" of a matrix. Let your mind think in pictures and sketch the essential concepts printed in each of the following windowpanes. Don't be concerned with your artistic ability. Use lines and stick figures to depict the concepts requested.

Consultation Card	Styling Books	Personal Portfolio
Photos	Digital Camera	Color Charts
Color Swatches	Mirror	Mannequin

7 ESSENTIAL EXPERIENCE

Topics to Avoid

In the space provided make a list of at least six topics that you should avoid discussing with clients. Then write a brief explanation as to why these topics would be inappropriate and list alternative topics that you might suggest if the client should bring up any of these.

Explanation and Alternative Topics:

_____

_____

_____

_____

_____

_____

_____

_____

_____

_____

_____

_____

_____

_____

_____

True or False

Circle the T for true or the F for false as applicable to the following statements to form a thorough review of Chapter 4: Communicating for Success.

T   F   **1.** A fundamental factor in human relations has to do with how secure we are feeling.

T   F   **2.** Communicate from your head; problem solve from your heart.

T   F   **3.** Show people you care by listening to them and trying to understand their point of view.

T   F   **4.** Effective human relations and communication skills build lasting client relationships, aid in your growth, and help prevent misunderstandings.

T   F   **5.** Communication is the act of effectively sharing information between two people, or groups of people, so that it is effectively understood.

T   F   **6.** To earn a client's trust and loyalty, you need to always approach a new client in a formal and reserved manner.

T   F   **7.** The client consultation is the written communication that determines the desired results.

T   F   **8.** The work and consultation area needs to be freshly cleaned and uncluttered.

T   F   **9.** Reflective listening is the process of repeating back to the client, in your own words, what you think she is telling you.

T   F   **10.** If a client doesn't fully realize that her choice in a service will not benefit her, it is your obligation to find a way to bluntly let her know.

T   F   **11.** The verbal communication with a client that is used to determine the client's desired results is called a client consultation.

ESSENTIAL REVIEW *continued*

T   F   **12.** A consultation with a first-time client should be scheduled at least 15 minutes prior to the actual appointment.

T   F   **13.** Record any formulations or products used, including the strength and any specific techniques followed, on the Rolodex.

T   F   **14.** When meeting a client for the first time, always introduce yourself.

T   F   **15.** The first step in the client consultation process is to ask the client what he/she likes least and most about his/her current look.

T   F   **16.** Encouraging a client to flip through photo collections and point out finished looks that he/she likes and why is called the show-and-tell step of the consultation.

T   F   **17.** It is important to counsel the client on salon and home maintenance commitments needed to keep the look as well as lifestyle limitations.

T   F   **18.** If a client arrives late, you should establish a precedent by refusing to complete the service under any circumstances.

T   F   **19.** If a client shows up at an incorrect time or day, politely explain his/her mistake and offer to reschedule them.

T   F   **20.** Never argue with a client or try to force your opinion on him/her.

T   F   **21.** Using unkind words or actions with regard to your colleagues is sometimes necessary.

T   F   **22.** Your job and your relationship with your clients are very specific: the goal is to advise and service clients with their beauty needs, and nothing more.

4

ESSENTIAL DISCOVERIES AND ACCOMPLISHMENTS

In the space below, jot some notes about what concepts of this chapter were hardest for you to understand or remember. Imagine finding yourself suddenly in the role of "teacher" and consider what you would tell your "students" about these difficult concepts. Share your Essential Discoveries with some of the other students in your class and ask if they are helpful to them. You may want to revise your notes based on good ideas shared by your peers. Under Accomplishments, list at least three things you have accomplished since your last entry that relate to your career goals.

Discoveries:

_____

_____

_____

_____

_____

_____

_____

_____

Accomplishments:

_____

_____

_____

_____

_____

INFECTION CONTROL: PRINCIPLES & PRACTICES

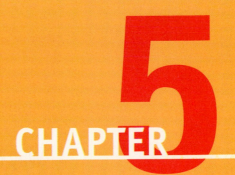

CHAPTER 5

A Motivating Moment: "It is amazing what ordinary people can do if they set out without preconceived notions."—Charles Kettering

ESSENTIAL OBJECTIVES

After studying this chapter and completing the Essential Companion components, you should be able to:

1. Understand state laws and rules.

2. List the types and classifications of bacteria.

3. List the types of disinfectants and how they are used.

4. Define hepatitis and HIV and explain how they are transmitted.

5. Describe how to safely clean and disinfect salon tools and equipment.

6. Explain the differences between cleaning, disinfection, and sterilization.

7. Discuss universal precautions and your responsibilities as a salon professional.

ESSENTIAL PRINCIPLES AND PRACTICES OF INFECTION CONTROL

Why do I need to know about the principles of infection control?

If you work in cosmetology or a related career field, you will come in contact with the public on a regular basis in a variety of ways. Understanding bacteriology, sterilization, and sanitation will make a big difference in how you protect yourself and your clients from the spread of infection or disease. There has never been a time in our history when the public has been more aware of how easily disease can be spread. Your clients' perceptions of you will be greatly improved if you convey both knowledge and concern about bacteria and the spread of disease.

There is an old saying that you never get a second chance to make a positive first impression. Nothing could be more appropriate for the first impressions you and your establishment make on the public. They will judge you by the cleanliness of the establishment where you work, by the cleanliness of your work station and implements, and by the neat, well-groomed image you present. Today's public demands that their doctors, dentists, optometrists, and beauty service professionals practice the highest levels of infection control and decontamination. So, if you want to build a solid, repeat clientele for the services in which you specialize, you will want to practice obvious sanitation and disinfection measures to build client confidence and trust in you. In addition, you must be able to take the necessary steps to protect yourself from infection by treating a client who may have an infectious disease that can't be identified by you.

What are the essential concepts of providing the safest possible environment using effective decontamination and infection control procedures?

As a professional in the cosmetology industry, you will need to understand the difference between nonpathogenic (helpful or harmless) and pathogenic (harmful) bacteria. You will need to know the various classifications of bacteria and how to identify each. It is essential that you develop an understanding of bacterial growth and reproduction, bacterial infections, other infectious agents, immunity, and acquired immune deficiency syndrome (AIDS).

As a successful licensee in the field of cosmetology or related discipline, you will need to know about both prevention and control. You need to understand that surfaces may be contaminated even if they appear clean; you will also need to know the steps necessary to make those surfaces germ free. You will learn procedures and products for sanitation and sterilization as well as disinfection and will gain knowledge about the tools and implements to accomplish both. The Occupational Safety and Health Administration (OSHA) plays an important role in the responsibilities each licensed establishment has to ensure a safe work environment both for workers and the public. By taking the approach known as universal precautions and following the same infection control practices with all clients, regardless of their health status, you are ensuring the best possible protection for you and the public.

INFECTION CONTROL: PRINCIPLES & PRACTICES

Mind Mapping

Mind mapping creates a free-flowing outline of material or information. Using the central or key point of *Staphylococci,* diagram the types of things staph is responsible for, sources of staph or how staph can be picked up, and symptoms of staph. Use terms, pictures, and symbols as desired. Using color will increase memory of the material.

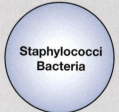

Staphylococci
Bacteria

2
ESSENTIAL EXPERIENCE

Match the following essential terms with their identifying terms or phrases.

_____	Bacteria	1. Lives and reproduces by penetrating cells.
_____	Pathogenic	2. Powerful tuberculocidal disinfectants.
_____	Infectious	3. Kills most, but not all, microorganisms on nonliving surfaces.
_____	Toxin	4. One-celled microorganisms.
_____	Virus	5. An organism that lives on another organism.
_____	Mitosis	6. Cleaning.
_____	Efficacy	7. Elimination of microbial life.
_____	Local infection	8. Contagious disease caused by the itch mite.
_____	Mildew	9. Harmful bacteria.
_____	Parasites	10. Can be spread from one person to another.
_____	Scabies	11. Poisonous substance.
_____	Sanitation	12. Cell division.
_____	Disinfection	13. Effectiveness of a solution to kill germs.
_____	Sterilization	14. Confined to a specific part of body.
_____	Phenolics	15. A type of fungus.

3
ESSENTIAL EXPERIENCE

Imagine that you own a professional establishment. You are committed to maintaining the highest levels of sanitation and client protection possible. Take a tour through your establishment and identify and list the areas in the salon that are most susceptible to pathogenic bacteria.

_____

_____

_____

_____

_____

_____

4

Word Scramble—Bacteriology

Scramble	Correct Word
aasseptir	_ _ _ _ _ _ _ _ _
	Clue: Require living matter for growth.
fsuoniceti	_ _ _ _ _ _ _ _ _ _
	Clue: Contagious.
aiarcetb	_ _ _ _ _ _ _ _
	Clue: Minute, one-celled vegetable microorganisms.
alcicyoocshpt	_ _ _ _ _ _ _ _ _ _ _ _ _
	Clue: Grow in bunches or clusters.
asseibc	_ _ _ _ _ _ _
	Clue: Caused by an itch mite.
cpnaiegoht	_ _ _ _ _ _ _ _ _ _
	Clue: Disease producing.
mrseg	_ _ _ _ _
	Clue: Also known as bacteria.
napnocnghieot	_ _ _ _ _ _ _ _ _ _ _ _ _
	Clue: Helpful or harmless.
calol fctnoiine	_ _ _ _ _ _ _ _ _ _ _ _ _ _
	Clue: Contains pus.
seborcim	_ _ _ _ _ _ _ _
	Clue: Also known as germs or bacteria.
ssriminagoorcm	_ _ _ _ _ _ _ _ _ _ _ _ _ _
	Clue: Bacteria are an example of this.
ucosaignto	_ _ _ _ _ _ _ _ _ _
	Clue: Spreads by contact.

4 ESSENTIAL EXPERIENCE *continued*

uicedsslpoi

_ _ _ _ _ _ _ _ _ _ _

Clue: Head lice.

bdnftsiieaelc

_ _ _ _ _ _ _ _ _ _ _ _ _

Clue: Item that can be disinfected.

ieaitnpsct

_ _ _ _ _ _ _ _ _ _

Clue: Chemical germicides for skin.

dcgnflaiiu

_ _ _ _ _ _ _ _ _

Clue: Capable of destroying fungus.

aaiiommnnftl

_ _ _ _ _ _ _ _ _ _ _ _

Clue: Body's response to injury or infection.

ttiisphea

_ _ _ _ _ _ _ _ _

Clue: Bloodborne virus.

oosurp

_ _ _ _ _ _

Clue: Absorbent.

belrtcalduucoi

_ _ _ _ _ _ _ _ _ _ _ _ _ _

Clue: Type of disinfectant.

5 ESSENTIAL EXPERIENCE

As in the game of Jeopardy, write questions which would be correctly answered.

Infection Control for $100.

1. Three types of potentially infectious microorganisms.

   _____

2. Also known as germs and can exist almost anywhere on the skin of the body, in water, air, decayed matter, secretions of body openings, on clothing, and beneath the nails.

   _____

3. Disease producing when they invade plant or animal tissue.

   _____

Infection Control for $200.

1. The life cycle of bacteria.

   _____

2. The stage in which microorganisms grow and reproduce.

   _____

3. Cells that are formed through mitosis.

   _____

Infection Control for $300.

1. Occurs when body tissues are invaded by disease-causing or pathogenic bacteria.

   _____

2. Bacteria normally carried by about a third of the population.

   _____

3. They are responsible for contagious diseases and conditions, such as head lice.

   _____

5

5

ESSENTIAL EXPERIENCE *continued*

Infection Control for $400.

1. The ability of the body to destroy bacteria that have gained entrance, and thus resist infection.

   _____

2. Something the body develops after it has overcome a disease, or through inoculation.

   _____

3. A disease that is transmittable by contact.

   _____

Infection Control for $500.

1. A person can be infected with this for many years without having symptoms.

   _____

2. It is transmitted through unprotected sexual contact, IV drug users sharing needles, and accidents with needles in health care settings.

   _____

3. It causes AIDS.

   _____

6 ESSENTIAL EXPERIENCE

Complete the following partial Safety and Health Inspection Report for your institution which is adapted from *Safety and Health in the Salon.* Write a brief explanation if an area is out of compliance.

Location: _____ Inspected by: _____ Date: _____

All Areas—Housekeeping and Sanitation

There is evidence the facility has been used for cooking or living quarters. ___ Yes ___ No

All areas are orderly, dusted, clean, sanitary, well-lighted, and rodent free. ___ Yes ___ No

Floors are swept clean and hair is swept up after each client service. ___ Yes ___ No

Windows, screens, and curtains are cleaned regularly. ___ Yes ___ No

Waste materials are deposited in a metal waste receptacle with a self-closing lid. ___ Yes ___ No

Waste receptacles are emptied regularly throughout the day. ___ Yes ___ No

All sinks and drinking fountains are cleaned regularly. ___ Yes ___ No

Separate or disposable drinking cups are provided for clients, employees, and students. ___ Yes ___ No

Hot and cold water faucets are clean and leakfree. ___ Yes ___ No

Toilets and washing facilities are clean and sanitary. ___ Yes ___ No

Toilet tissue, paper towels, and pump-like antiseptic liquid soap are provided. ___ Yes ___ No

Door handles are cleaned regularly. ___ Yes ___ No

Food is stored separately from clinic products. ___ Yes ___ No

Eating and drinking are done on sanitary surfaces separate from chemical handling or where services are being performed. ___ Yes ___ No

Work area is appropriately ventilated for services provided; fans, humidifiers, and exhaust and ventilation systems are cleaned regularly. ___ Yes ___ No

5

6 ESSENTIAL EXPERIENCE *continued*

Floors are free of water or other substances that could cause a slip, trip, or fall. ___ Yes ___ No

MSDS are available for all chemicals used in the clinic. ___ Yes ___ No

All chemicals are properly stored and all containers are properly labeled. ___ Yes ___ No

Appropriate personal protective equipment (eye protection, gloves, dust and organic vapor masks, etc.) is available and used according to manufacturer's directions and salon policy. ___ Yes ___ No

Washing machine provides water temperature of at least 160 degrees Fahrenheit. ___ Yes ___ No

Hospital-grade tuberculocidal disinfecting solution and instructions are available for cleaning combs, brushes, plastic capes, and other materials as required. ___ Yes ___ No

Emergency Precautions and First Aid

Emergency phone numbers are posted where they can be readily found in an emergency. ___ Yes ___ No

Fire evacuation procedures are posted. ___ Yes ___ No

First aid kits are readily accessible with necessary supplies. ___ Yes ___ No

First aid kit is periodically inspected and replenished as needed. ___ Yes ___ No

Emergency eye wash bottles are provided where chemical handling is done and where chemical services are provided. ___ Yes ___ No

There is ready access to a sink with tempered water to completely flush the eyes from hazardous materials. ___ Yes ___ No

Exit and warning signs (biohazard, fire door, flammable or toxic chemicals) are posted where appropriate. ___ Yes ___ No

7 ESSENTIAL EXPERIENCE

Word Search—Decontamination

Word	Clue
alcohol	There are three widely used forms.
antiseptics	These can kill bacteria but are not disinfectants.
asymptomatic	Showing no symptoms or signs of infection.
contaminant	Causes contamination.
contaminated	Surfaces which look clean, may still be this.
decontamination	There are three levels of this.
disinfectants	Kill microbes on nonporous surfaces.
disinfection	Controls microorganisms on nonporous surfaces.
household bleach	Sodium hypochlorite.
MSDS	Provides pertinent information about ingredients.
OSHA	This is part of the United States Department of Labor.
QUATS	Safe and fast-acting disinfectant.
sanitation	Lowest level of decontamination.
sterilization	Most effective decontamination.

After finding the appropriate word from the above clues, locate the word in the following word search puzzle.

```
C A N T I S E P T I C S A A N Q S A
O L S A N I T A T I O N U Q U H T S
N D O X Y F O B Z O X D B A O C E Y
T Q E H S O L Z J Q V I T U H O R M
A A W C O O F F U Y Y S S X G N I P
M A R D O C L F R O P E U K E T L T
I H C J M N L T G Y H C U Q S A I O
N L R Y C M T A M O K C Z A P M Z M
A R I C Y T F A L S W V K N Y I A A
T P C G B R O D M M D U I Y D N T T
E N E N Y S B S W I S F L E M A I I
D M Q T H L L A P W N D X Y S N O C
V T I A E N W Q C S X A S J S T N D
S H P A Q N Y D C E P N T J O A A L
F A C B V A L A F C D B H I A E H N
C H K I R J L K D S A R H K O R H H
M E J N O I T C E F N I S I D N V D
D I S I N F E C T A N T S L H D J P
```

5

ESSENTIAL REVIEW

Using the following words, fill in the blanks below to form a thorough review of
Chapter 5: Infection Control

acquired immunity	hepatitis B	outer covering	scabies
boils	HIV	parasites	spherical spores
contagious	immunity	pathogenic	*streptococci*
daughter cells	local	pimples	syphilis
diphtheria	mitosis	pneumonia	twelve
disinfectant	natural	protoplasm	virus
eleven	nonpathogenic	pus	viruses
general	one-celled	round-shaped	

1. Staphylococci are pus-forming organisms that grow in clusters and cause
   _____ and _____ .

2. A _____ infection is indicated by a boil or pimple and contains
   pus.

3. Organisms that live on other living organisms and do not give anything in
   return are known as _____ .

4. The body's ability to destroy bacteria that have gained entrance is called
   _____ .

5. Bacteria are _____ vegetable microorganisms found nearly
   everywhere.

6. _____ is a fluid created by tissue inflammation.

7. Infectious diseases and conditions such as _____ should never
   be treated in a school or salon, but referred to a physician.

8. _____ are infectious microorganisms smaller than bacteria and
   capable of infesting almost all plants and animals.

9. The body develops _____ after it has overcome a disease or
   through inoculation.

10. A person can be infected with _____ for many years without
    having symptoms.

ESSENTIAL REVIEW *continued*

11. _____ organisms are harmful and produce disease.

12. A _____ infection results when the bloodstream carries the bacteria or virus and their toxins to all parts of the body.

13. When bacteria grow and reach their largest size, they divide and split into two new cells. The division is called _____ and the new cells formed are called _____ .

14. Immunity against disease can be _____ or acquired.

15. When a disease becomes _____ it spreads from one person to another.

For the remainder of the review, circle the correct answer to each question.

16. Any surface that is not free of dirt, hair, or microbes is _____ .
    a) sterilized   b) contaminated
    c) sterile   d) disinfected

17. The three levels of decontamination are sterilization, disinfection, and _____.
    a) washing   b) dusting
    c) sweeping   d) sanitation

18. The methods of sterilization include high-pressure steam or _____ .
    a) dry heat autoclave b) gaseous formaldehyde
    c) liquid antiseptic   d) dry sanitation

19. Substances that kill microbes on contaminated tools and other nonporous surfaces are _____ .
    a) antiseptics   b) tablets
    c) disinfectants   d) liquids

20. Disinfectants must be registered with the _____ .
    a) DOE   b) EPA
    c) APE   d) DOL

ESSENTIAL REVIEW *continued*

21. Federal law requires manufacturers to provide product information on the
_____ .

a) MSDS
b) MDSD
c) SMDS
d) MSSD

22. The Occupational Safety and Health Administration was created as part of the _____ .

a) DOJ
b) DOE
c) DOL
d) DOA

23. Most QUATS disinfect implements within _____ minutes.

a) 1–3
b) 4–5
c) 6–8
d) 10

24. If salon implements come into contact with blood, they should be cleaned and immersed in _____ .

a) quaternary ammonium compounds
b) phenolic disinfectants
c) sodium hypochlorite
d) EPA registered disinfectant

25. The third and lowest level of decontamination is known as _____ .

a) disinfection
b) sterilization
c) sanitation
d) immunization

ESSENTIAL DISCOVERIES AND ACCOMPLISHMENTS

In the space below, jot some notes about what concepts of this chapter were hardest for you to understand or remember. Imagine finding yourself suddenly in the role of "teacher" and consider what you would tell your "students" about these difficult concepts. Share your Essential Discoveries with some of the other students in your class and ask if they are helpful to them. You may want to revise your notes based on good ideas shared by your peers. Under Accomplishments, list at least three things you have accomplished since your last entry that relate to your career goals.

Discoveries:

_____

_____

_____

_____

_____

_____

_____

_____

Accomplishments:

_____

_____

_____

_____

GENERAL ANATOMY AND PHYSIOLOGY

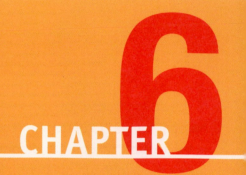

CHAPTER **6**

A Motivating Moment: "Don't go where the path may lead, go instead where there is no path and leave a trail."—Ralph Waldo Emerson

ESSENTIAL OBJECTIVES

After studying this chapter and completing the Essential Companion components, you should be able to:

1. Explain the importance of anatomy and physiology to the cosmetology profession.

2. Describe cells, their structure, and their reproduction.

3. Define *tissue* and identify the types of tissues found in the body.

4. Name the 10 body systems and explain their basic functions.

ESSENTIAL ANATOMY AND PHYSIOLOGY

Why do I need to know about cells and the anatomy and physiology of the body when I just want to do hair?

As you do hair and perform all the other services you are qualified and trained to perform, almost without exception, you will be affecting the bones, muscles, and nerves of the body. Therefore, it is essential that you understand the basic anatomy and physiology of the body to perform all those services safely and effectively. If you think about it, you will realize that when you cut hair, you must understand the contours of the head and its bone structure. When you apply makeup, you must perform contouring based on the bone and muscle structure of the face. When giving a scalp treatment, you need to know about the circulatory system in order to achieve maximum stimulation of the scalp, and so forth.

Even though you may not consider studying about anatomy and physiology as the most exciting or glamorous part of your training, it is clearly an integral part of your training and will contribute significantly to your effectiveness and success. Certainly your knowledge in this key area will gain your clients' trust and confidence in your credibility.

ESSENTIAL CONCEPTS

What do I need to learn about cells and anatomy and physiology to be more effective as a cosmetologist?

The cell is the basic structure from which all other body structures are made. You will want to develop a comfortable knowledge about cell growth and metabolism. You will want a basic knowledge of each of the main systems of the body and of tissue. Once you've gained information about how each organ or system functions and its purpose, you can be more effective in the services you provide.

1

ESSENTIAL EXPERIENCE

Mind Map—Cell Development

Mind mapping creates a free-flowing outline of material or information. The central or key point is located in the center. The key point of this mind map is process of development from a basic cell to the various types of tissue to forming organs and developing systems. Using color will increase the mind's retention of the material. Keep your mind open and uncluttered, and don't worry about where a line or word should go as the organization of the map will usually take care of itself.

2
ESSENTIAL EXPERIENCE

Organs

Label each of the organs indicated in the diagram of a human body. State the purpose of each part of the body in the space provided. You may need to refer to your school's reference library for assistance.

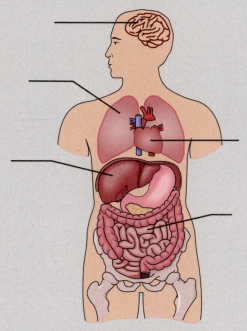

Brain: _____

_____

Heart: _____

_____

Lungs: _____

_____

Liver: _____

_____

Digestive tract: _____

_____

3

ESSENTIAL EXPERIENCE

Matching Exercise—Body Systems

Match each of the following essential terms with its definition.

_____ Circulatory

_____ Digestive

_____ Endocrine

_____ Excretory

_____ Integumentary

_____ Muscular

_____ Nervous

_____ Reproductive

_____ Respiratory

_____ Skeletal

1. Duct glands and ductless glands.

2. The process of converting food into a form that can be assimilated by the body.

3. The physical foundation or framework of the body.

4. Situated in the chest cavity, protected by the ribs.

5. Covers, shapes, and supports the skeleton; produces all body movements.

6. Made up of the skin and its various accessory organs.

7. Organs for reproducing.

8. Controls and coordinates the functions of all the other systems and makes them work harmoniously and efficiently.

9. Kidneys, liver, skin, intestines, and lungs; purifies the body by eliminating waste matter.

10. Controls the steady circulation of the blood.

4

Matching Exercise A—The Muscular System

Match each of the following essential terms with its definitions.

Word	Clue
_____ Frontalis	1. Enables closing of eye.
_____ Orbicularis oculi	2. Controls shoulder blades.
_____ Pectoralis	3. Assists in swinging of arms.
_____ Serratus anterior	4. Rotates arms.
_____ Biceps	5. Assists in breathing and raising arms.
_____ Trapezius	6. Raises the eyebrows; wrinkles forehead.
_____ Triceps	7. Lifts forearm and flexes elbow.
_____ Extensors	8. Extends arm outward.
_____ Flexors	9. Extends forearm.
_____ Latissimus dorsi	10. Allow the wrist to bend.
_____ Deltiod	11. Straighten wrist, hand, and fingers.

5

ESSENTIAL EXPERIENCE

Matching Exercise B—The Muscular System

Match each of the following essential terms with its definitions.

Word	Clue
_____ Pronators	**1.** Draw fingers together.
_____ Supinator	**2.** Draws the scalp backward.
_____ Abductors	**3.** Covers, shapes, and supports skeleton.
_____ Muscular system	**4.** Coordinates opening and closing of mouth.
_____ Occipitalis	**5.** Rotates palm upward.
_____ Aponeurosis	**6.** Separate the fingers.
_____ Masseter	**7.** Lowers jaw and lip.
_____ Adductors	**8.** Lowers and rotates the head.
_____ Platysma	**9.** Turn hands inward.
_____ Sternocleidomastoideus	**10.** Draws eyebrow down and wrinkles forehead.
_____ Corrugator	**11.** Connects occipitalis and frontalis.

6

ESSENTIAL EXPERIENCE

Bones and Muscles of the Cranium

Using a shaved mannequin or a Styrofoam head block, draw a line from the center front "hairline" to the center nape. On side one, draw in and label the bones of the head. On side two, draw in and label the muscles of the head. (Refer to your text for assistance.) In the absence of a mannequin or head block, use the diagrams below.

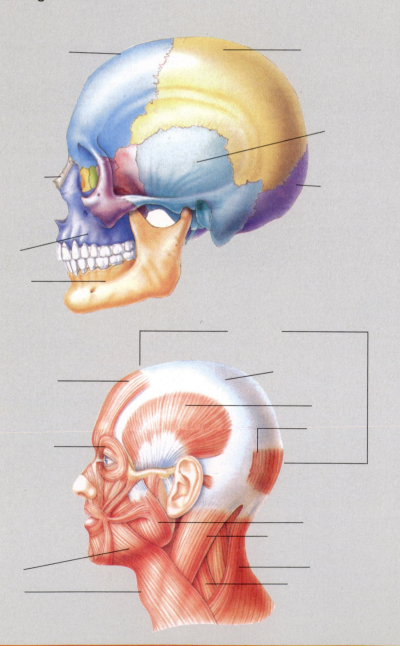

7

ESSENTIAL EXPERIENCE

Word Search A—Circulatory System

After determining the correct word from the clues provided, locate the words in the word search puzzle.

Word	Clue
_____	Thick-walled muscular and elastic tubes that carry pure blood from the heart to the capillaries.
_____	Right- or left-upper, thin-walled chambers of the heart.
_____	The nutritive fluid circulating through the circulatory system.
_____	Minute, thin-walled blood vessels that connect smaller arteries to veins.
_____	The main source of blood supply to the head, face, and neck.

```
B J Z Z Z N Y L R A H C V G O W S L
Z H E S N U M U C P D C M J U E J D
V N Y M G T H O H C U G J Z I C L C
Z K G U U G G A Q T L E K R A F I X
Z J J S D I O O H E Z I E P C C N D
U G C R Z I R A I R H T I Y V T T H
G R U A S A T T T Y R L A Y N J T M
C F L E T P M O A A L Y V Z X E P E
Z P A D G G Y J R A V H P N L U G X
S T E J H J P R R A B I A X C H P H
E T M P J P X I I S C V W R V T W C
O V X W N P E X F O F N T D K Y K B
U T Y S B S H T W E C L O Q R Q P A
U X Y P C L U R J M J Y E M H S V W
L O E K C B N G S N J Z E S M D U L
Y G O G I B L M V L A F C F H O Q X
N Z P G Q M P D B P V S F A S Q C D
S R A C I T C U M C N L H D O O L B
```

6

8

Word Search B—Circulatory System

After determining the correct word from the clues provided, locate the words in the word search puzzle.

Word	Clue
_____	A clear, yellowish fluid that carries waste and impurities away from the cells.
_____	The fluid part of the blood in which the red and white blood cells and blood platelets flow.
_____	Blood circulation that goes from the heart to the lungs to be purified.
_____	Artery that supplies the thumb side of the arm and the back of the hand.
_____	Artery that supplies the little finger side of the arm and the palm of the hand.
_____	Allow blood to flow in only one direction.
_____	The circulatory system.
_____	Thin-walled blood vessels that are less elastic than arteries.
_____	Right or left lower thick-walled chambers of the heart.

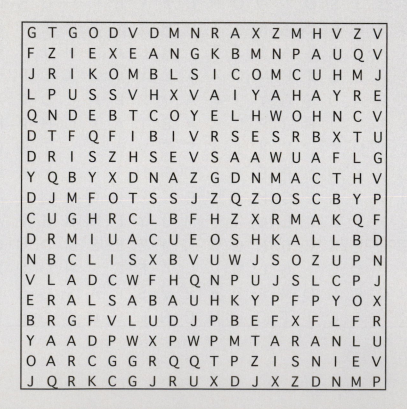

```
G T G O D V D M N R A X Z M H V Z V
F Z I E X E A N G K B M N P A U Q V
J R I K O M B L S I C O M C U H M J
L P U S S V H X V A I Y A H A Y R E
Q N D E B T C O Y E L H W O H N C V
D T F Q F I B I V R S E S R B X T U
D R I S Z H S E V S A A W U A F L G
Y Q B Y X D N A Z G D N M A C T H V
D J M F O T S S J Z Q Z O S C B Y P
C U G H R C L B F H Z X R M A K Q F
D R M I U A C U E O S H K A L L B D
N B C L I S X B V U W J S O Z U P N
V L A D C W F H Q N P U J S L C P J
E R A L S A B A U H K Y P F P Y O X
B R G F V L U D J P B E F X F L F R
Y A A D P W X P W P M T A R A N L U
O A R C G G G R Q Q T P Z I S N I E V
J Q R K C G J R U X D J X Z D N M P
```

ESSENTIAL REVIEW

Complete the following review of Chapter 6: General Anatomy and Physiology by circling the correct answer to each question.

1. The uppermost and largest bone of the arm is the _____ .
   a) humerus
   b) radius
   c) ulna
   d) metacarpus

2. The structure of the cell found in the center, which plays an important part in cell reproduction, is the _____ .
   a) nucleus
   b) centrosome
   c) cell membrane
   d) nucleolus

3. The involuntary muscles that function automatically are called

   _____ .
   a) striated
   b) striped
   c) nonstriated
   d) cardiac

4. To grow and thrive, the cell must receive an adequate supply of food, oxygen, and _____ .
   a) toxins
   b) poisons
   c) pressure
   d) water

5. A group of cells of the same kind are _____ .
   a) organs
   b) tissues
   c) systems
   d) groups

6. The artery that supplies the back of the head up to the crown is the

   _____ .
   a) supraorbital
   b) occipital
   c) facial artery
   d) posterior auricular

7. The process of building up larger molecules from smaller ones is called

   _____ .
   a) anabolism
   b) homeostasis
   c) catabolism
   d) secretion

8. The small bone on the thumb side of the forearm is the _____ .
   a) humerus
   b) radius
   c) ulna
   d) metacarpus

9. The muscle that produces the contour of the front and inner side of the upper arm is called the _____ .
   a) cardiac
   b) tricep
   c) bicep
   d) epicranius

10. The epicranius consists of two parts, the frontalis and the _____ .
   a) aponeurosis
   b) occipito-frontalis
   c) corrugator
   d) occipitalis

11. Structures designed to accomplish a specific function are _____ .
   a) organs
   b) tissues
   c) systems
   d) groups

12. Cells are made up of a colorless, jellylike substance called _____ .
   a) nucleolus
   b) nucleus
   c) protoplasm
   d) centrosome

13. The study of the structure of the body and what it is made of is _____ .
   a) physiology
   b) histology
   c) anatomy
   d) osteology

14. The _____ system changes food into soluble form, suitable for use by the cells of the body.
   a) endocrine
   b) respiratory
   c) excretory
   d) digestive

15. The wrist, or _____ , is a flexible joint composed of eight small, irregular bones.
   a) metacarpus
   b) ulna
   c) carpus
   d) digits

16. The _____ vascular system consists of the heart and blood vessels for the circulation of the blood.
   a) lymph
   b) circulatory
   c) lymphatic
   d) blood

17. The process of breaking down larger substances or molecules into smaller ones is _____ .
   a) anabolism
   b) homeostasis
   c) catabolism
   d) secretion

18. The study of the minute structural parts of the body, such as tissues, hair, nails, sweat glands, and oil glands is _____ .
    a) physiology
    b) histology
    c) anatomy
    d) osteology

19. The fingers, or _____ , consist of three phalanges in each finger, and two in the thumb, totaling 14 bones.
    a) metacarpus
    b) ulna
    c) carpus
    d) digits

20. The scientific study of bones, their structure, and functions is

    _____ .
    a) physiology
    b) histology
    c) anatomy
    d) osteology

21. The elastic, bony cage that serves as a protective framework for the heart, lungs, and other internal organs is the _____ .
    a) sternum
    b) clavicle
    c) scapula
    d) thorax

22. The part of the cell that contains food materials necessary for growth, reproduction, and self-repair is the _____ .
    a) cytoplasm
    b) centrosome
    c) nucleolus
    d) cell membrane

23. The _____ system's function is to produce all movements of the body.
    a) circulatory
    b) skeletal
    c) muscular
    d) nervous

24. The physical foundation of the body is the _____ system.
    a) circulatory
    b) skeletal
    c) muscular
    d) nervous

25. Voluntary muscles that are controlled by will are called _____ .
    a) striated
    b) smooth
    c) nonstriated
    d) cardiac

26. What bone forms the lower back part of the cranium?
    a) parietal
    b) temporal
    c) frontal
    d) occipital

27. The part of the muscle that moves is the _____ .
    a) origin
    b) belly
    c) insertion
    d) middle

28. The _____ system is made up of the skin and its various accessory organs.
    a) endocrine
    b) excretory
    c) integumentary
    d) reproductive

29. The muscle that completely surrounds the margin of the eye socket is the

    _____ .

    a) corrugator
    b) orbicularis oculi
    c) procerus
    d) orbicularis oris

30. The _____ vertebrae form the top part of the spinal column located in the neck region.
    a) cervical
    b) thorax
    c) hyoid
    d) thoracic

31. What bone forms the forehead?
    a) parietal
    b) temporal
    c) frontal
    d) occipital

32. The muscle that forms a flat band around the upper and lower lip is the

    _____ .

    a) caninus
    b) mentalis
    c) orbicularis oris
    d) buccinator

33. A broad muscle that extends from the chest and shoulder to the side of the chin is the _____ .
    a) pectoralis
    b) serratus anterior
    c) platysma
    d) supinators

34. The _____ turn the hand outward and palm upward.
    a) pectoralis
    b) serratus anterior
    c) platysma
    d) supinators

ESSENTIAL REVIEW *continued*

35. The muscle that straightens the wrist, hand, and fingers to form a straight line is the _____ .
- a) opponent
- b) adductor
- c) extensors
- d) abductor

36. The _____ muscles draw the fingers together.
- a) opponent
- b) adductor
- c) extensors
- d) abductor

37. The _____ system controls and coordinates the functions of all the other systems and makes them work harmoniously.
- a) circulatory
- b) skeletal
- c) muscular
- d) nervous

38. The _____ and the temporalis coordinate in opening and closing the mouth and are referred to as chewing muscles.
- a) triangularis
- b) risorius
- c) zygomaticus
- d) masseter

39. There are three main divisions of the nervous system: the central, the _____ , and the autonomic nervous systems.
- a) peripheral
- b) sympathetic
- c) parasympathetic
- d) brain

40. The _____ assists in breathing and in raising the arm.
- a) pectoralis
- b) serratus anterior
- c) platysma
- d) supinators

41. The _____ nerve supplies all the fingers of the hand.
- a) ulnar
- b) radial
- c) median
- d) digital

42. The lower thick-walled chambers of the heart are the left and right _____ .
- a) atrium
- b) ventricle
- c) auricle
- d) valves

ESSENTIAL REVIEW *continued*

43. Minute, thin walled blood vessels that connect the smaller arteries to the veins are the _____ .
    - a) arteries
    - b) veins
    - c) capillaries
    - d) blood

44. The _____ system is situated within the chest cavity, which is protected on both sides by the ribs.
    - a) endocrine
    - b) respiratory
    - c) excretory
    - d) digestive

45. _____ circulation is the blood circulation from the heart throughout the body and back again to the heart.
    - a) Systemic
    - b) Plasma
    - c) Pulmonary
    - d) Platelet

46. The fluid part of the blood in which the red and white blood cells and blood platelets flow is _____ .
    - a) lymph
    - b) corpuscles
    - c) leukocytes
    - d) plasma

47. A clear yellowish fluid that carries waste and impurities away from the cells is known as _____ .
    - a) lymph
    - b) corpuscles
    - c) leukocytes
    - d) plasma

48. The artery that supplies the crown and side of the head is the _____ .
    - a) parietal
    - b) transverse
    - c) temporal
    - d) frontal

49. The system that purifies the body by eliminating waste material is the _____ system.
    - a) endocrine
    - b) respiratory
    - c) excretory
    - d) digestive

50. The collar bone that joins the sternum and scapula is called the _____ .
    - a) humerus
    - b) ulna
    - c) radius
    - d) clavicle

ESSENTIAL DISCOVERIES AND ACCOMPLISHMENTS

In the space below, jot some notes about what concepts of this chapter were hardest for you to understand or remember. Imagine finding yourself suddenly in the role of "teacher" and consider what you would tell your "students" about these difficult concepts. Share your Essential Discoveries with some of the other students in your class and ask if they are helpful to them. You may want to revise your notes based on good ideas shared by your peers. Under Accomplishments, list at least three things you have accomplished since your last entry that relate to your career goals.

Discoveries:

_____

_____

_____

_____

_____

_____

_____

_____

Accomplishments:

_____

_____

_____

_____

SKIN STRUCTURE & GROWTH

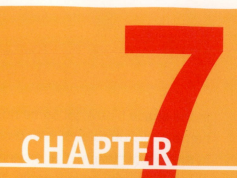

CHAPTER 7

A Motivating Moment: "Work as though you would live forever, and live as though you would die today."—Og Mandino

ESSENTIAL OBJECTIVES

After studying this chapter and completing the Essential Companion components, you should be able to:

1. Describe the structure and composition of the skin.

2. List the functions of the skin.

ESSENTIAL HISTOLOGY OF THE SKIN

Why do I need to learn about the skin structure and growth when I really want to specialize as a hair designer?

You actually do not need the level of knowledge that a scientist would have on this subject matter. However, a thorough knowledge of the underlying structures of the skin, nails, and hair will benefit you in your role as a professional cosmetologist. The skin is the largest and one of the most important organs of the body. Therefore, it becomes one of the most important subjects about which you need to know because so many cosmetology services deal directly with the skin—whether you are providing hair and/or scalp service, facial or skin care service, or nail care service. All those services require you to come in direct contact with clients' skin. Knowledge of the skin will help you achieve the best possible results when providing these treatments, while also providing the safest care for your clients. Remember, happy clients come back and often bring their friends with them. That means greater financial success for you.

ESSENTIAL CONCEPTS

What do I need to know about the structure and growth of the skin in order to perform professionally as a cosmetologist?

Skin care is one of the fasting growing areas of the cosmetology industry. By thoroughly analyzing the functions, structure, and components of the skin, you will better understand how the skin actually works. You will learn that with proper care, your skin and the skin of your clients can remain young and look radiant for many years. You will need to understand how the skin is nourished and how the various glands affect the functions of the skin.

1 ESSENTIAL EXPERIENCE

Analysis of the Epidermis

Using the chart below, analyze the structure of the epidermis. The first column lists each layer; in the second column, explain what quality this structure adds to the skin; and in the third column, list the purpose of the layer.

Layer	Composition	Purpose
Stratum corneum		
Stratum lucidum (clear layer)		
Stratum granulosum (granular layer)		
Stratum spinosum		
Stratum germinativum (basal cell layer)		

2
ESSENTIAL EXPERIENCE

Skin Layer Reconstruction

Using various household items or food products, create a model cross-section of the following layers of the skin:

Basal cell layer (stratum germinativum)

Stratum spinosm

Stratum granulosum

Stratum lucidum

Stratum corneum

Papillary layer

Reticular layer

Subcutaneous tissue

Either paste your items in the space provided or use poster board to make a larger model. (Hint: Items you might use include Rice Krispies, corn flakes, Fruit Loops, honey, a slice of bread, and/or a soft flour tortilla.) Once you've built your model, compare it to Figure 7-2 in your textbook.

3 ESSENTIAL EXPERIENCE

Matching

Match each of the following essential functions of the skin with its description.

_____ Protection

_____ Sensation

_____ Heat regulation

_____ Excretion

_____ Secretion

_____ Absorption

1. Sebum or oil that lubricates the skin, keeping it soft and pliable. Oil also keeps hair soft. Emotional stress can increase the flow of sebum.

2. Perspiration from the sweat glands is eliminated through the skin. Water lost through perspiration takes salt and other chemicals with it.

3. The skin shields the body from injury and bacterial invasion. The outermost layer of the epidermis is covered with a thin layer of sebum, thus rendering it waterproof. It is resistant to wide variations in temperature, minor injuries, chemically active substances, and many forms of bacteria.

4. Through the nerve endings, the skin responds to heat, cold, touch, pressure, and pain. When nerve endings are stimulated, a message is sent to the brain that directs you to respond accordingly.

5. An ingredient or chemical can enter the body through the skin and influence it to a minor degree. Fatty materials, such as lanolin creams, are taken in largely through hair follicles and sebaceous gland openings.

6. The skin protects the body from the environment by maintaining a constant internal body temperature of about 98.6 degrees Fahrenheit. As changes occur in the outside temperature, the blood and sweat glands make necessary adjustments and the body is cooled by the evaporation of sweat.

4

ESSENTIAL EXPERIENCE

Crossword Puzzle

Word	Clue
Collagen	Fibrous protein that gives the skin form and strength.
Dermatologist	Physician engaged in the science of treating the skin, its structures, functions, and diseases.
Dermatology	Medical branch of science that deals with the study of skin.
Dermis	Underlying or inner layer of the skin.
Elastin	Protein base similar to collagen; forms elastic tissue.
Epidermis	Outermost layer of the skin.
Basal	Layer of skin referred to as the stratum germinativum.
Spiny	Layer of skin referred to as the stratum spinosum.
Granular	Layer of skin referred to as the stratum granulosum.
Stratum lucidum	Clear, transparent layer of skin.
Papillary	Cuticle layer of the dermis.
Reticular	The deeper layer of the dermis.
Subcutaneous	Fatty layer found below the dermis.

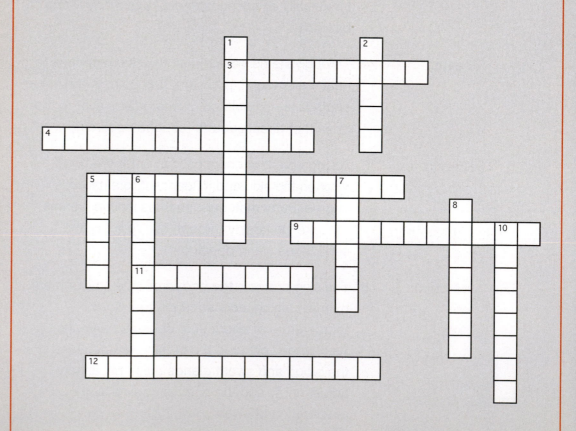

ESSENTIAL REVIEW

Complete the following review of Chapter 7: Skin Structure and Growth by circling the correct answer to each question.

1. The clear layer of the epidermis, consisting of small transparent cells, is the _____ .
   a) stratus lucidum
   b) stratum granulosum
   c) stratum corneum
   d) stratum germinativum

2. The basal cell layer, composed of several layers of different shaped cells, is the _____ .
   a) stratum lucidum
   b) stratum granulosum
   c) stratum corneum
   d) stratum germinativum

3. The outermost layer of the skin is the _____ .
   a) dermis
   b) subcutaneous
   c) epidermis
   d) adipose

4. The dermis is about _____ times thicker than the epidermis.
   a) 10
   b) 25
   c) 35
   d) 40

5. Which layer of the dermis houses the nerve endings that provide the body with the sense of touch?
   a) papillary
   b) reticular
   c) corium
   d) cutis

6. Which layer of the skin contains numerous blood vessels, lymph vessels, nerves, sweat glands, oil glands, and hair follicles as well as arrector pili muscles?
   a) subcutaneous
   b) dermis
   c) adipose
   d) epidermis

7. The underlying or inner layer of the skin is the _____ .
   a) dermis
   b) subcutaneous
   c) epidermis
   d) adipose

8. What is secreted by the sudoriferous glands?
   a) perspiration
   b) blood
   c) odor
   d) sebum

ESSENTIAL REVIEW *continued*

9. What controls the excretion of sweat?
   a) circulatory system
   b) nervous system
   c) excretory system
   d) respiratory system

10. A fatty layer found below the dermis is the _____ .
    a) dermis
    b) subcutaneous tissue
    c) epidermis
    d) true skin

11. The skin responds to heat, cold, touch, pressure, and pain through stimulation of the _____ .
    a) internal body temperature
    b) sudoriferous glands
    c) sensory nerve endings
    d) body fluid absorption

12. No oil glands are found here.
    a) palms
    b) face
    c) forehead
    d) scalp

13. Vitamin _____ is an antioxidant that can help prevent certain types of cancers and has been shown to improve the skin's elasticity and thickness.
    a) A
    b) B
    c) C
    d) D

14. The best source for vitamin _____ is sunlight.
    a) A
    b) B
    c) C
    d) D

15. Drinking pure water sustains the health of the cells, aids in the elimination of toxins and waste, helps regulate body temperature, and aids in proper _____ .
    a) osmosis
    b) metabolism
    c) digestion
    d) congestion

16. The secretory nerves, which are distributed to the sweat and oil glands of the skin, are part of the _____ .
    a) circulatory system
    b) autonomic nervous system
    c) excretory system
    d) respiratory system

ESSENTIAL REVIEW *continued*

17. _____ supplies nutrients and oxygen to the skin.
   a) Lymph   b) Nerves
   c) Blood   d) Sweat

18. Vitamin _____ helps fight against and protect the skin from the harmful effects of the sun's rays.
   a) A   b) C
   c) D   d) E

19. Vitamin _____ is vitally important in fighting the aging process and promotes the production of collagen.
   a) A   b) C
   c) D   d) E

20. Small epidermal structures with nerve endings that are sensitive to touch and pressure are _____ .
   a) tactile corpuscles   b) sudoriferous glands
   c) subcutaneous tissue   d) sebaceous glands

ESSENTIAL DISCOVERIES AND ACCOMPLISHMENTS

In the space below, jot some notes about what concepts of this chapter were hardest for you to understand or remember. Imagine finding yourself suddenly in the role of "teacher" and consider what you would tell your "students" about these difficult concepts. Share your Essential Discoveries with some of the other students in your class and ask if they are helpful to them. You may want to revise your notes based on good ideas shared by your peers. Under Accomplishments, list at least three things you have accomplished since your last entry that relate to your career goals.

Discoveries:

_____

_____

_____

_____

_____

_____

_____

_____

_____

_____

Accomplishments:

_____

_____

_____

_____

_____

NAIL STRUCTURE & GROWTH

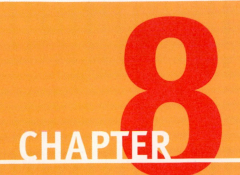

A Motivating Moment: "My great concern is not whether you have failed, but whether you are content with your failure."—Abraham Lincoln

ESSENTIAL OBJECTIVES

After studying this chapter and completing the Essential Companion components, you should be able to:

1. Describe the structure and composition of nails.

2. Discuss how nails grow.

ESSENTIAL NAIL STRUCTURE AND GROWTH

I am going to be a cosmetologist; why do I need to learn about the structure of the nail?

That's a very good question. The fact is that the structure and growth of the nail is certainly not the most glamorous portion of your training in cosmetology, but could be one of the most essential. More infections are spread through the nails and hands than any other area of the body. To give clients professional and responsible service, you must learn about the structure and function of the nail. You must know when it is safe to work on a client and when they must be referred to a doctor. So, learning about the structure and growth of the nail is extremely relevant to your future success and well-being.

ESSENTIAL CONCEPTS OF NAIL STRUCTURE AND GROWTH, DISEASES, AND DISORDERS

What do I need to know about the nail, its structure, and growth in order to provide quality manicuring and pedicuring services?

You will need to recognize that the condition of the nail may actually reflect the general health of the whole body. You need to understand the structure of the nail and also the structures surrounding the nail. Once you understand how the nail grows, you will be better equipped to recognize the malformations, disorders, and irregularities that your clients may bring to the salon. When you've gained that knowledge, you can proceed confidently with appropriate nail services knowing that you and your client are not at risk. Refer to Chapter 24 for more information on Nail Diseases and Disorders.

1

ESSENTIAL EXPERIENCE

Label the parts of the nail on the front view and cross-section diagrams using the terms listed below. Note that some essential terms may be used more than once.

Nail bed	Eponychium
Free edge	Hyponychium
Matrix	Ligament
Lunula	Nail fold
Nail plate	Nail grooves
Cuticle	

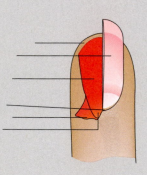

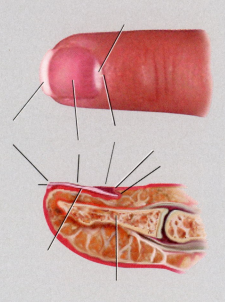

Matching Exercise—Structures Surrounding the Nail

Match the following essential terms with their identifying phrases or definition.

_____ Cuticle

_____ Eponychium

_____ Hyponychium

_____ Matrix

_____ Nail grooves

_____ Nail bed

_____ Nail folds

_____ Lunula

_____ Ligament

_____ Free edge

_____ Nail plate

1. Slits or furrows at either side of the nail, upon which the nail moves as it grows.

2. The dead colorless tissue attached to the nail plate.

3. The slightly thickened layer of skin that lies underneath the free edge of the nail plate.

4. Normal skin that surrounds the nail plate.

5. The portion of the living skin on which the nail plate sits.

6. The living skin at the base of the nail plate covering the matrix area.

7. Where the natural nail is formed.

8. The most visible and functional part of the nail.

9. The part of the nail plate that extends over the tip of the finger.

10. A tough band of fibrous tissue that connects bones or holds an organ in place.

11. The lighter color shows the true color of the matrix.

ESSENTIAL EXPERIENCE

Windowpane

Window paning is the process of transferring key elements, points, or steps in a lesson into visual images that are hand sketched into the squares or "panes" of a matrix. Let your mind think in pictures and sketch the essential concepts printed in each of the following windowpanes. Don't be concerned with your artistic ability. Use lines and stick figures to depict the concepts requested for the various shapes of the nail.

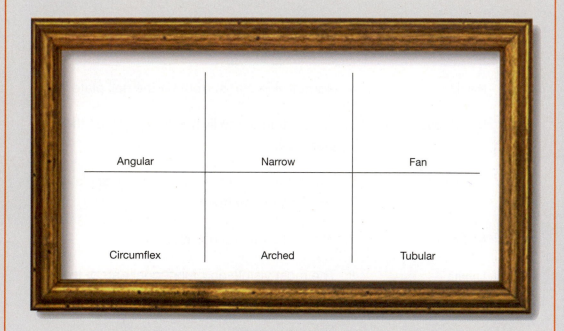

Angular	Narrow	Fan
Circumflex	Arched	Tubular

4

Word Search

After identifying the appropriate word from the clues listed below, locate the word in the following word search puzzle.

Word	Clue
_____	Composed mainly of keratin.
_____	Visible part of the matrix that extends from underneath the living skin.
_____	Where the natural nail is formed.
_____	Attaches the nail bed and matrix bed to the underlying bone.
_____	Dead colorless tissue attached to the nail plate.
_____	Helps guide the nail plate along the nail bed as it grows.

```
O V L E Z M F H S C S N U B G N S C
G F T U J P S Q Q X B Y F N X O U S
Q T E J N E V V P S A H Q N L T A L
R A Y M V U P A F V P X E I I Y Y U
N G B X I F L I H A A Z A C Z X O I
U B T J X Z H A T E W N L B D C L V
E M N E T K J P K H L E X D X L K U
A C F S M G X X M A E F B H T X A P
H T S N M Q Q G R O T L Z W V O A D
T P K J D S B U V S X N I Q A Y J W
S Y Y G M E T P D E L J E U Q G N V
J Z A A T A Z V S T J N I M M P Q X
I N C B N K T J I U N D E X A F H U
K T R E A Y P H T M K Z C O Q G M P
M P T D G S J W P G I O C J C T I J
P I D A F A Q F W O O O B Q P G E L
D U J X U O J X S W R R X I R T A M
F R C X A T A Y S Q B A M M F V A M
```

8

ESSENTIAL REVIEW

Complete the following review of Chapter 8: Nail Structure and Growth by circling the correct answer to each question.

1. The nail is an appendage of the skin and is part of the _____ .
   a) circulatory system
   b) skeletal system
   c) integumentary system
   d) muscular system

2. A healthy nail may look dry and hard, but it actually has a water content of between _____ .
   a) 10 and 20 percent
   b) 15 and 25 percent
   c) 20 and 30 percent
   d) 25 and 35 percent

3. The matrix is composed of matrix cells that produce the nail _____ .
   a) lunula
   b) plate
   c) grooves
   d) mantle

4. The nail bed is supplied with many nerves and is attached to the nail plate by a thin layer of tissue called the _____ .
   a) bed epithelium
   b) hyponychium
   c) nail grooves
   d) eponychium

5. The visible part of the matrix that extends from underneath the living skin is the _____ .
   a) lunula
   b) hyponychium
   c) matrix
   d) eponychium

6. The slits or furrows on the sides of the nail on which it moves as it grows is called the _____ .
   b) nail folds
   b) ligaments
   c) nail plate
   d) nail grooves

7. In an adult, the nail grows at an average of _____ inch per month.
   a) 1/10
   b) 1/16
   c) 1/4
   d) 3/8

ESSENTIAL REVIEW *continued*

8. Ordinary replacement of a natural nail takes about _____ .

   a) 2 to 4 months   b) 3 to 5 months
   c) 4 to 6 months   d) 5 to 7 months

9. Toenails take _____ months to a year to be fully replaced.

   a) 4   b) 6
   c) 7   d) 9

ESSENTIAL DISCOVERIES AND ACCOMPLISHMENTS

In the space below, jot some notes about what concepts of this chapter were hardest for you to understand or remember. Imagine finding yourself suddenly in the role of "teacher" and consider what you would tell your "students" about these difficult concepts. Share your Essential Discoveries with some of the other students in your class and ask if they are helpful to them. You may want to revise your notes based on good ideas shared by your peers. Under Accomplishments, list at least three things you have accomplished since your last entry that relate to your career goals.

Discoveries:

_____

_____

_____

_____

_____

_____

_____

_____

_____

_____

Accomplishments:

_____

_____

_____

_____

_____

PROPERTIES OF THE HAIR & SCALP

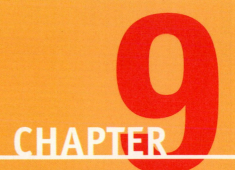

A Motivating Moment: "Keep in mind that the true measure of an individual is how he treats a person who can do him absolutely no good."—Ann Landers

ESSENTIAL OBJECTIVES

After studying this chapter and completing the Essential Companion components, you should be able to:

1. Name and describe the structures of the hair root.

2. List and describe the three layers of the hair shaft.

3. Describe the three types of side bonds in the cortex.

4. List the factors that should be considered in a hair analysis.

5. Describe the process of hair growth.

6. Discuss the different types of hair loss and their causes.

7. Describe the various options for hair loss treatment.

8. Recognize hair and scalp disorders commonly seen in the salon and school, and know which can be treated by cosmetologists.

ESSENTIAL PROPERTIES OF THE HAIR AND SCALP

How will knowing about the underlying theory of the properties of the hair and scalp help me to be a more successful cosmetologist?

Men and women of all ages want healthy, attractive hair. As a licensed cosmetology professional, you will be called upon to advise all your clients on the best care and treatment of their hair both inside and outside the professional establishment. In order to provide the best possible counsel to your clients, you must have a thorough understanding of the hair and how it can be damaged. Hair is composed of different layers which are responsible for specific hair qualities. It will be essential for you to be able to analyze the client's hair, determine what type of damage the hair has experienced, and properly prescribe corrective treatments. None of these tasks will be possible without your knowledge of the various properties of the hair and scalp.

ESSENTIAL CONCEPTS

What are the key concepts a professional cosmetologist must understand in order to properly analyze a client's hair and prescribe appropriate corrective treatments?

Trichology is the technical term for the study of hair. As you proceed through your study of trichology, you will gain important insights into how the hair is distributed over the body and the scalp. You will learn that hair is composed chiefly of the protein called keratin and there are two principal parts of hair, the hair root and the hair shaft. As well as understanding the structure of hair, you will learn how it grows. Most importantly, however, you will learn to use the senses of sight, touch, hearing, and smell to analyze the condition of a client's hair. Key elements in hair analysis include several hair qualities, including texture, porosity, and elasticity. You will also determine that effective scalp manipulation on a regular basis will stimulate the muscles and nerves of the scalp as well as increase the blood circulation in the scalp area.

Another important area of awareness is that of hair loss and how it affects over 63 million people in the United States. This particular malady can range from the most common type of hair loss, androgenetic alopecia, which is a result of progressive shrinking or miniaturization of certain scalp follicles, to postpartum alopecia, which is a temporary hair loss after pregnancy. The professional cosmetologist must also be able to identify various diseases and disorders of the hair and scalp since they are not allowed to treat certain conditions that must be referred to a medical professional for treatment.

1

ESSENTIAL EXPERIENCE

Hair Purpose

In your own words, explain the purpose of the two main types of hair found on the body: vellus and terminal hair.

Vellus: _____

_____

_____

_____

_____

_____

Terminal: _____

_____

_____

_____

_____

_____

2

ESSENTIAL EXPERIENCE

Hair Follicle Structure

Using the following key, please label the cross-section of the hair.

arrector pili	epidermis	sebaceous or oil glands
bulb	hair follicle	
dermal papilla	hair root	

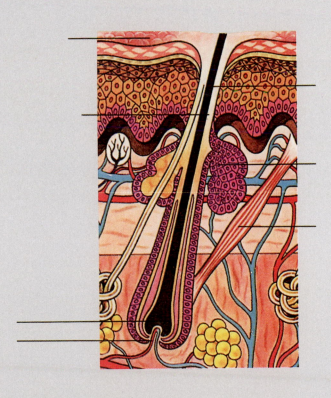

3

Hair Structure

Using colored pencils or crayons, draw a cross-section of the hair and follicle depicting and labeling each of the following categories.

- Cortex
- Cuticle
- Medulla

4 ESSENTIAL EXPERIENCE

Hair Replacement and Growth

Hair growth occurs in cycles. Each complete cycle has three phases that are repeated over and over again throughout life. The three phases are anagen, catagen, and telogen. In your own words, please explain each phase.

Anagen: _____

_____

_____

_____

_____

Catagen: _____

_____

_____

_____

Telogen: _____

_____

_____

_____

5

ESSENTIAL EXPERIENCE

Directional Hair Growth

Find two individuals with distinct and different hair growth patterns. Using the following head outlines, diagram the growth patterns.

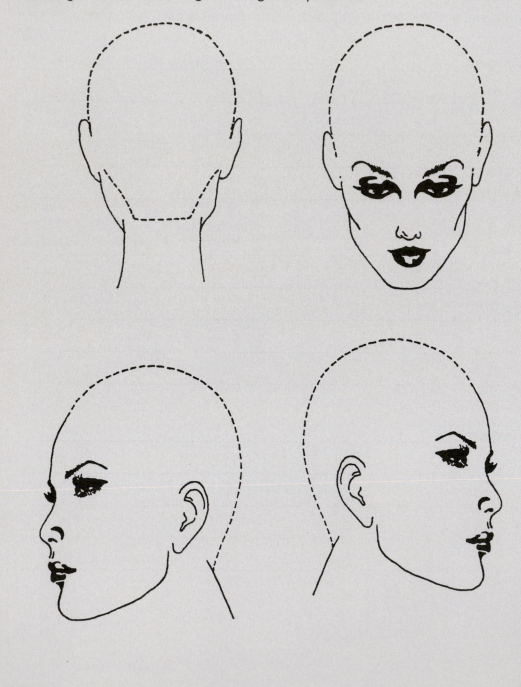

6

ESSENTIAL EXPERIENCE

Word Search—Properties of the Hair and Scalp

After determining the correct words from the clues provided, locate the words in the word search puzzle.

Word	Clue
_____	Abnormal hair loss.
_____	Growth phase in the hair cycle in which new hair is created.
_____	The lowest area or part of a hair strand.
_____	The technical term for gray hair.
_____	Inflammation of the subcutaneous tissue caused by *Staphylococci*.
_____	Transitional phase of hair growth.
_____	Outermost layer of hair.
_____	The number of hairs per square inch on the scalp.
_____	Chemical side bond that joins the sulfur atoms of two neighboring cysteine amino acids to create cystine.
_____	The ability of the hair to stretch and return to its original length.
_____	Tubelike depression, or pocket, in the skin or scalp that contains the hair root.
_____	Combined with crinium, it's the technical term for brittle hair.
_____	Innermost layer of hair.
_____	Technical term for beaded hair.
_____	Dandruff.
_____	The ability of the hair to absorb moisture.
_____	The part of the hair structure found below the skin surface.
_____	Skin disease caused by the "mite."
_____	Dry, sulfur-yellow, cuplike crusts on the scalp in tinea favosa or favus.
_____	The portion of the hair that projects beyond the skin.
_____	The degree of coarseness or fineness of the hair.
_____	Ringworm.
_____	Hair that forms in a circular pattern, as on the crown.

6

ESSENTIAL EXPERIENCE *continued*

```
D C A D B Z J H Y A C W H O R L A E
E E A L I P A K W C T J T B A L L A
B I N T O S V V F P V O P L U C E N
N A B S A P U N T P A S B T I N E P
K O U F I G E L J Q N Z U T I G H I
E Q L X P T E C F H S C U T A Y G T
F U B U W N Y N I I S C X N T D Q Y
E T F G Y V C H T A D I A I N O V R
E F S S L P Z U Z F R E S H H L K I
L R P F M R K C A H O O B U Z I X A
A A G W J Q W L T S R L S O R I B S
S G D T J R L E E O T S L H N A E I
T I D E N U L I P R W E C I A D T S
I L R F D I T X T W H N X A C F I M
C I D E N I U W D G R I K T B L T D
I T M O N R W C U W Y S M C U I E O
T A M A K C M N S T I R O O T R E Y
Y S C C A R B U N C L E C W S Y E S
```

Crossword Puzzle—Properties of the Hair and Scalp

Word	Clue
Dermal papilla	Small, cone-shaped area located at the base of the hair follicle.
Arrector pili	Involuntary muscle in the base of the hair follicle.
Sebaceous	Oil glands of the skin.
Sebum	Oily substance that lubricates the hair and skin.
Cortex	The middle layer of hair.
Amino	Acids that are linked together end to end.
Peptide	Chemical bond that links amino acids together.
Hydrogen	A weak physical side bond easily broken.
Melanin	Pigment in the cortex, gives natural color to hair.
Stream	Hair flowing in the same direction.
Cowlick	Tuft of hair that stands straight up.
Vellus	Short, fine, downy hair.
Terminal	Long hair found on scalp, legs, arms, and bodies.
Telogen	Resting phase of hair cycle.
Hypertrichosis	Abnormal hair growth.
Trichoptilosis	Technical term for split ends.
Monilethrix	Technical term for beaded hair.

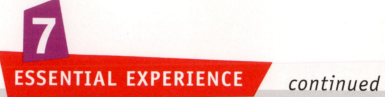
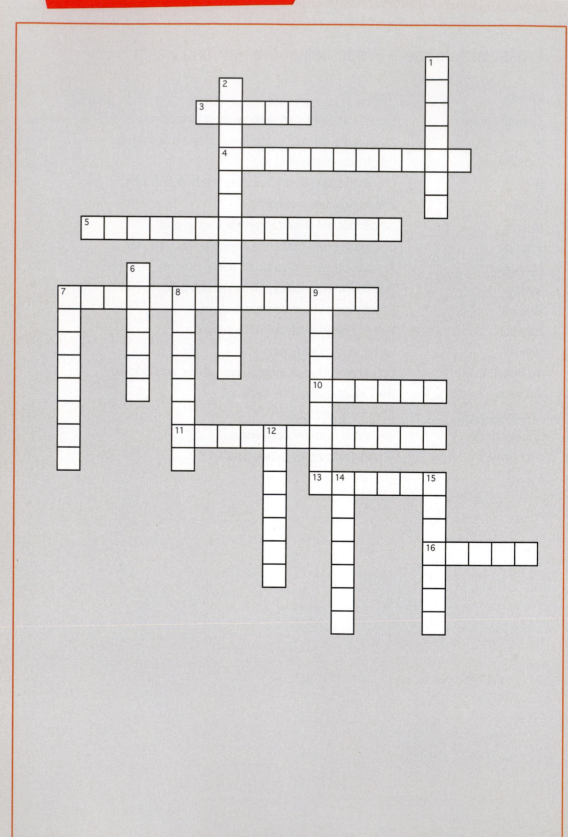

8 ESSENTIAL EXPERIENCE

Grouping Properties of the Hair and Scalp by Category

Place the following terms or procedures into the appropriate category in the chart.

alopecia areata	dermal papilla	pediculosis	tinea capitis
anagen	elasticity	capitis	simplex
androgenetic	fenasteride	pityriasis	tinea
alopecia	fine	pityriasis capitis	tinea favosa
arrector pili	follicle	simplex	trichorrhexis
bulb	fragilitas crinium	pityriasis	nodosa
canities	hair root	steatoides	trichoptilosis
catagen	hair stream	porosity	vellus hair
cortex	hypertrichosis	postpartum	whorl
cowlick	keratin	alopecia	
cuticle	medulla	scabies	
dandruff	Minoxidil	telogen	
density	monilethrix	texture	

Hair Distribution, Composition, and Structure:

_____

Hair Growth:

_____

Hair Analysis:

_____

Hair Loss:

_____

Hair Disorders:

_____

Scalp Disorders:

_____

9

ESSENTIAL REVIEW

Using the following words, fill in the blanks below to form a thorough review of Chapter 9, Properties of the Hair and Scalp. Words or terms may be used more than once.

80%	cortex	hypertrichosis	sebum
90%	cuticle	keratinization	simplex
acidic	dandruff	miniaturized	*Staphylcocci*
alkaline	dermal papilla	monilethrix	steatoides
amino acids	disulfide	nodular	swelling
androgenetic	elasticity	one-half	terminal
alopecia	eumelanin	oval	three
arrector pili	follicle	pediculosis	topical
boil	hair bulb	polypeptide	trichology
brittle	hair root	porosity	trichoptilosis
canities	hair shaft	round	unpigmented
carbuncle	hair stream	scabies	vellus
cells	healthy diet	scutula	
chemicals	hydrogen	sebaceous	

1. The study of the hair is technically called _____ .

2. The technical term for the hair found on the face is known as _____ .

3. One basic requisite for healthy hair is a _____ .

4. Full-grown human hair is divided into two principal parts which are known as the hair root and the _____ .

5. The two most common types of _____ infections are furuncles and carbuncles.

6. The technical term for hair found on the head is _____ hair.

7. A tube-like depression or pocket in the skin or scalp that encases the hair root is called the _____ .

8. The thickened, club-shaped structure that forms the lower part of the hair root is known as the _____ .

ESSENTIAL REVIEW *continued*

9. The small involuntary muscle attached to the underside of the hair follicle is called the _____ .

10. Fear or cold causes the _____ to contract, which makes the hair stand up straight, giving the appearance of "goose bumps."

11. Oil glands which consist of a sac-like structure in the dermis are the _____ glands.

12. An oily substance secreted from the sebaceous glands which keeps the skin surface soft and supple is _____ .

13. Hair is composed of cells arranged in _____ layers.

14. The outermost layer of the hair is called the _____ .

15. The cuticle layer of the hair can be raised by _____ .

16. The _____ is the middle layer of the hair which gives elasticity.

17. The _____ is that portion of the hair that projects beyond the skin.

18. The _____ is that portion of the hair that is located below the surface of the scalp.

19. The small cone-shaped area located at the base of the follicle is the _____ .

20. The average growth of healthy hair on the scalp is about _____ inch per month.

21. Hair flowing in the same direction is known as _____ .

22. Cross-sections of straight hair tend to be _____ .

23. Hair is composed of protein that grows from cells originating within the hair follicle. They mature in a process called _____ .

24. Cross-sections of extremely curly hair tend to be _____ .

ESSENTIAL REVIEW *continued*

25. Qualities by which human hair is analyzed are texture, density, _____ , and _____ .

26. The ability of the hair to stretch and return to its original form is _____ .

27. The ability of the hair to absorb moisture is known as _____ .

28. Hair is composed of protein that grows from _____ originating within the hair follicle.

29. Hair is approximately _____ protein.

30. The technical term for the most common type of hair loss is _____ .

31. Hair protein is made up of long chains of _____ , which are made up of elements.

32. A long chain of amino acids linked by peptide bonds is called a _____ chain.

33. A _____ bond is a physical side bond that is easily broken by water or heat.

34. Minoxidil is a _____ medication applied to the scalp twice daily to stimulate hair growth.

35. The technical term for gray/unpigmented hair is _____ .

36. Salt bonds are easily broken by strong _____ or _____ solutions.

37. An abnormal development of hair on areas of the body that normally bear only downy hair is known as _____ or hirsutism.

38. The technical term for split hair ends is _____ .

39. Trichorrhexis nodosa, or knotted hair, is the dry, brittle condition including formation of _____ swellings along the hair shaft.

ESSENTIAL REVIEW   *continued*

40. The technical term for beaded hair is _____ , which may be improved with scalp and hair treatments.

41. Fragilitas crinium is the technical term for _____ hair that may split at any part of its length.

42. A _____ bond joins the sulfur atoms of two neighboring amino acids.

43. Pityriasis is the medical term for _____ .

44. Two different types of melanin are _____ and pheomelanin.

45. The two principal types of dandruff include pityriasis capitis _____ (the dry type) and pityriasis _____ (the greasy or waxy type).

46. Honeycomb ringworm is characterized by dry, sulfur-yellow, cup-like crusts on the scalp called _____ .

47. _____ is a highly contagious, animal parasitic skin disease caused by the itch mite.

48. A contagious condition caused by the head louse is _____ capitis.

49. A furuncle, or _____ , is an acute localized bacterial infection of a hair follicle.

50. A _____ is the result of an acute staphylococci infection and is larger than a furuncle.

ESSENTIAL DISCOVERIES AND ACCOMPLISHMENTS

In the space below, jot some notes about what concepts of this chapter were hardest for you to understand or remember. Imagine finding yourself suddenly in the role of "teacher" and consider what you would tell your "students" about these difficult concepts. Share your Essential Discoveries with some of the other students in your class and ask if they are helpful to them. You may want to revise your notes based on good ideas shared by your peers. Under Accomplishments, list at least three things you have accomplished since your last entry that relate to your career goals.

Discoveries:

_____
_____
_____
_____
_____
_____
_____
_____
_____
_____

Accomplishments:

_____
_____
_____
_____
_____

BASICS OF CHEMISTRY

A Motivating Moment: "Never measure the height of a mountain until you have reached the top. Then you will see how low it was."—Dag Hammarskjold

ESSENTIAL OBJECTIVES

After studying this chapter and completing the Essential Companion components, you should be able to:

1. Explain the difference between organic and inorganic chemistry.

2. Discuss the different forms of matter: elements, compounds, and mixtures.

3. Explain the difference between solutions, suspensions, and emulsions.

4. Explain pH and the pH scale.

5. Describe oxidation and reduction (redox) reactions.

Why is a basic knowledge of chemistry important to my career as a cosmetologist?

When you think about it, chemistry has an important role in every product you use, from the water you use to shampoo hair, to the cosmetics applied when giving a facial, to the chemicals you apply to hair in styling or in chemical reformation. Many of the services you will provide actually change the hair, skin, and nails chemically as well as physically. Therefore, it is essential that you have a good working knowledge of chemistry in order to provide the safest and most effective services to your clients.

What do I need to know about basic chemistry in order to be successful and more effective as a professional cosmetologist?

Like anatomy and physiology, chemistry may be a somewhat scary subject to you. Think of it this way: chemistry is simply the study of matter, its composition, structure, and properties, and the changes matter may undergo. You know that matter is anything that occupies space and has weight. Organic chemistry deals with all substances in which carbon is present. That, of course, includes animals, plants, petroleum, soft coal, natural gas, and many artificially prepared substances. Most will burn, but cannot be liquefied, even though they will dissolve inorganic solvents.

Inorganic chemistry, on the other hand, is the branch of chemistry that deals with all substances that do not contain carbon, such as water, air, iron, lead, minerals, and iodine. These are substances that will not burn and are usually soluble in water. Now, your goal in training as a cosmetologist is not to become a scientist, but to develop a comfort level with the basics and ability to discuss chemistry in relation to your profession. This will increase your credibility significantly with your clients, especially during the consultation process.

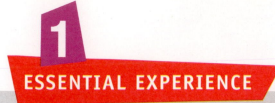

Organic Versus Inorganic Chemistry

Use your knowledge of the difference between organic and inorganic substances to gather at least 10 items in each category. List your items in the space provided and explain what makes them either organic or inorganic.

Organic	Inorganic

2

ESSENTIAL EXPERIENCE

Product Research

Research a variety of shampoo and conditioning products available in your school, at local supply stores, or at home. Use the chart below to track your findings.

Product Name	Key Ingredients	Purpose of Each Ingredient	Prescribed for Which Hair Type?

3

ESSENTIAL EXPERIENCE

Matter

In the space below, list examples of how matter can change form. Be specific. For example, when you melt an ice cube (a solid), it becomes water (a liquid), and when you boil it, it becomes steam (a gas). Not all your examples will include taking on all three forms.

_____

_____

_____

_____

_____

_____

_____

_____

_____

_____

_____

_____

_____

4 ESSENTIAL EXPERIENCE

Elements

An element is the basic unit of all matter. It is composed of a single part or unit and cannot be reduced to a more simple substance. There are 90 naturally occurring elements. Each element is identified by a letter symbol. The symbols for each element can be obtained by referring to the Periodic Table of Elements found in almost any chemistry textbook. Numbers are used with the elements to indicate how many parts are found in the substance. In the chart below, list the symbols for each substance and then explain its composition. (See the example for water.)

Substance	Symbol	Composition
Water	H_2O	Two parts hydrogen and one part oxygen
Ammonia		
Hydrogen Peroxide		
Nitric Acid		
Sodium Hydroxide		
Sodium Chloride		
Hydrogen		
Sulfur		
Nitrogen		
Oxygen		
Carbon		
Iron		
Lead		
Silver		

5
ESSENTIAL EXPERIENCE

Litmus Paper Testing

Obtain a variety of products and test their acidity and alkalinity using litmus paper. List the products you are testing below and state the results. Also, brush one piece of litmus paper with hydrogen peroxide, then brush one-half of the litmus paper with a hair color product. You will actually be able to see the oxidation process take place.

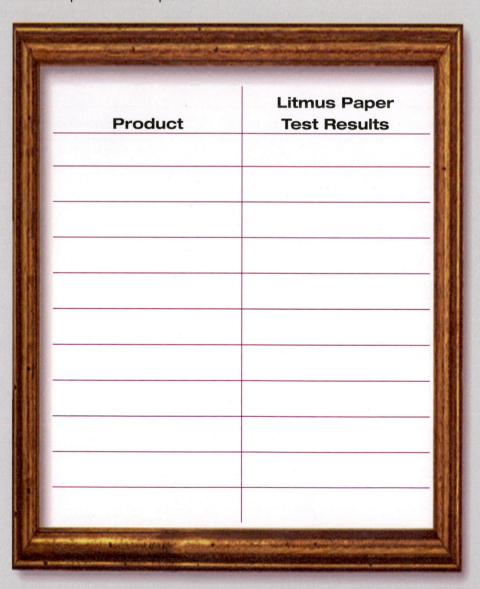

Product	Litmus Paper Test Results

6
ESSENTIAL EXPERIENCE

Crossword Puzzle

Word	Clue
Alkanolamines	Substances used to neutralize acids.
Emulsion	Mixture of two or more immiscible substances.
Exothermic	Chemical reaction that produces heat.
Glycerin	Sweet, colorless, oily substance used as a moisturizing ingredient.
Ionization	The separation of an atom or molecule into positive and negative ions.
Miscible	Capable of being mixed with another liquid.
Molecule	Two or more atoms joined chemically.
Redox	Contraction for reduction-oxidation.
Reduction	The subtraction of oxygen from, or the addition of hydrogen to.
Solute	The substance that is dissolved in a solution.
Solvent	The substance that dissolves the solute to form a solution.
Volatile	Easily evaporating.

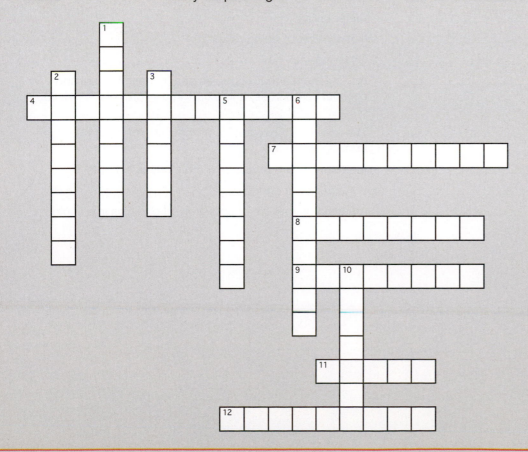

ESSENTIAL EXPERIENCE

Word Search

After determining the correct words from the clues provided, locate the words in the word search puzzle.

Word | **Clue**

_____ Solution having a pH below 7.

_____ Solution having a pH above 7.

_____ Colorless gas with pungent odor, composed of hydrogen and nitrogen.

_____ The smallest particle of an element that retains the properties of that element.

_____ Science that deals with the composition, structures, and properties of matter.

_____ Rapid oxidation of a substance.

_____ Chemical combination of two or more atoms of different elements.

_____ The simplest form of matter.

_____ Water loving.

_____ Not capable of being mixed.

_____ Oil loving.

_____ Any substance that occupies space, has physical and chemical properties, and exists in the form of a solid, liquid, or gas.

_____ The addition of oxygen to, or the subtraction of hydrogen from, a substance.

_____ A stable mixture of two or more mixable substances.

_____ Surface-active agent.

_____ An unstable mixture of undissolved particles in a liquid.

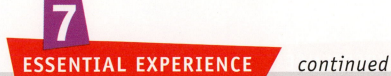

7

ESSENTIAL EXPERIENCE *continued*

```
S U R F A C T A N T R O C J Y S A I
J S P Y N O I T A D I X O T O T S M
A M K N H F H F V V P E N L O X O M
C M D J K G W K F E E U M Q W I I
U O M V X I B L N P M T C O V E A S
B Q M O Y G K R V E I I T P D U Y C
L F E B N K A A L O L A C Y O V A I
W N A L U I I E N I D P Z M D Y U B
V D A Y Y S A K H V L P I O B R C L
J Z R R X R T P U C Y U H Q A T I E
R X K C Z R O I D B C B V E E S L P
Z J N Z E R C A O N I W T T Y I I A
O F Z T D J J J F N U L C O X M H C
Q X T Y Q J F P A P A O A P H E P M
I A H L T G G T T C S C P K H H O R
M D Y F I K X X Q D L J I M L C P G
Y F D E Y R P S H M Y Z Y D O A I X
T K I O A N O I S N E P S U S C L D
```

8 ESSENTIAL EXPERIENCE

Matching Exercise

Match the following essential terms with their identifying phrases or definition.

_____ Chemical change

_____ Acid

_____ Ammonia

_____ Physical change

_____ Atom

_____ Glycerin

_____ Chemistry

_____ Ionization

_____ Redox

_____ Silicone

1. Special type of ingredients used in hair conditioners and as a water-resistant lubricant for the skin.

2. A sweet, colorless, odorless, oily substance used as a moisturizing agent.

3. The separation of an atom or molecule into positive and negative ions.

4. Chemical reaction in which the oxidizing agent is reduced and the reducing agent is oxidized.

5. A change in the form or physical properties of a substance without the formation of a new substance.

6. A change in the chemical and physical properties of a substance by a chemical reaction that creates a new substance.

7. The smallest particle of an element that retains the properties of that element.

8. A colorless liquid with a pungent odor composed of hydrogen and nitrogen.

9. Science that deals with the composition, structures, and properties of matter.

10. Having a pH below 7.

ESSENTIAL REVIEW

Using the words provided, fill in the blanks below to form a thorough review of
Chapter 10: Basics of Chemistry. Words or terms may be used more than once or
not at all.

acid	density	liquids	physical
alkali	element	matter	solvents
atom	emulsions	miscible	surfactant
chemical	hydrophilic	molecule	suspension
chemistry	inorganic	organic	volatile organic
compound	lipophilic	oxidizing	compounds

1. A solution with a pH less than 7 has an _____ pH; and a
   solution with a pH higher than 7 has an _____ pH.

2. A _____ change refers to a change in the form
   of a substance, without the formation of a new substance. A
   _____ change is when a new substance is formed.

3. A _____ is a substance that acts as a bridge to allow oil and
   water to mix or emulsify.

4. _____ are substances containing carbon which evaporate
   quickly and easily.

5. An _____ is the smallest particle of an element that is
   capable of showing the properties of an element.

6. Anything that occupies space is defined as _____ .

7. _____ are formed when two or more immiscible substances,
   such as oil and water, are united with the aid of a binder.

8. _____ chemistry is the branch of chemistry that deals with all
   substances that do not contain carbon.

9. Matter exists in three forms: solids, _____ , and gases.

10. _____ chemistry is the branch of chemistry that deals with all
    substances in which carbon is present.

11. _____ agents are substances that readily release oxygen.

12. _____ liquids are mutually soluble, meaning they can be
    mixed into stable solutions.

ESSENTIAL REVIEW *continued*

13. _____ are any substances that are able to dissolve another substance.

14. Surfactant molecules have two ends: _____ and _____ .

15. A _____ is an unstable mixture of undissolved particles in liquid.

16. The basic unit of all matter is an _____ .

17. The science that deals with the composition, structure, and properties of matter is _____ .

18. Two or more atoms that are joined together chemically form a _____ .

19. When a substance is made up of two or more different elements chemically joined, it is a _____ .

ESSENTIAL DISCOVERIES AND ACCOMPLISHMENTS

In the space below, jot some notes about what concepts of this chapter were hardest for you to understand or remember. Imagine finding yourself suddenly in the role of "teacher" and consider what you would tell your "students" about these difficult concepts. Share your Essential Discoveries with some of the other students in your class and ask if they are helpful to them. You may want to revise your notes based on good ideas shared by your peers. Under Accomplishments, list at least three things you have accomplished since your last entry that relate to your career goals.

Discoveries:

_____

_____

_____

_____

_____

_____

_____

_____

_____

Accomplishments:

_____

_____

_____

_____

BASICS OF ELECTRICITY

 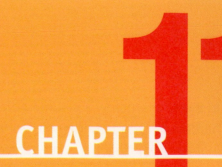

A Motivating Moment: "Now is a gift. That's why it is called the present. To be fully enjoyed, it must be unwrapped from the mistakes and guilt of the past and the worries of the future."—Unknown

ESSENTIAL OBJECTIVES

After studying this chapter and completing the Essential Companion components, you should be able to:

1. Define the nature of electricity and the two types of electrical currents.

2. Define electrical measurements.

3. Understand the principles of electrical equipment.

4. Describe electrical modalities used in cosmetology.

5. Explain electromagnetic radiation and the visible spectrum of light.

6. Describe the types of light therapies and their benefits.

ESSENTIAL ELECTRICITY

Why is a basic knowledge of electricity important to my career as a cosmetologist?

Electricity is the primary source of energy needed, literally, to run the world and the salon where you will work. Electricity is essential for controlling and maintaining the professional environment in every professional establishment. It is responsible for such things as lighting, ventilation, temperature, and possibly even the hot water you will use. Electricity must be used intelligently and safely. As a professional, you must know how it works in order to maintain a safe environment for yourself, your coworkers, and your clients.

Electricity is critical in the salon for use with blow dryers, curling irons, lotion heaters, wax heaters, facial equipment, cash registers, telephones, computers, nail drills, and much more. While it is not necessary for you to become an electrical engineer, it is important that you have a working knowledge of how electricity is created and how it can be used safely in the salon.

What do I need to know about basic electricity in order to be successful and more effective as a professional cosmetologist?

You need to be aware of the two types of electricity, how it is measured, and safety devices pertaining to electricity. You will need to have a working knowledge of the various types of currents that are used in the equipment found in the salon. It might help you to think of electricity in terms of the *flow* of an electric current. As a flow, an electric current is similar to a flow of water. It has a direction, requires a pathway, and can be stopped and started. While the flow of water can actually help create energy, the electric current *is* a flow of energy. It is this passage of energy that gives electricity powers than can be therapeutic or, if handled incorrectly, potentially dangerous and destructive.

The pathway for an electric current flowing through an appliance is called a circuit, which means that the current makes a kind of circle from its source through a conductor and back to its source again. If the current flows in a circuit constantly in one direction, it is called a *direct current* (DC). Most battery-operated devices use direct current. However, most appliances linked by a wall plug to a regional power system use *alternating current* (AC). In alternating current, the current changes direction in a circuit back and forth many times a second.

The flow of electricity can be stopped by simply breaking the circuit—by flipping a switch. When the switch is "on," the circuit is completed and electricity can flow. When the switch is "off," the circuit is broken and electricity cannot flow.

1

ESSENTIAL EXPERIENCE

Matching Exercise—Electrical Measurements

Match the following essential terms with its definition or identifying term.

_____ Volt

1. Measurement of how much electric energy is being used in 1 second.

_____ Amp

2. 1/1000 of an ampere.

_____ Milliampere

3. The unit of measurement for the amount of current running through a wire

_____ Ohm

4. Unit for measuring the pressure that forces the electric current forward.

_____ Watt

5. The electricity in your house is measured in this manner.

_____ Kilowatt

6. This unit measures the resistance of an electric current.

2

ESSENTIAL EXPERIENCE

Safety of Electrical Equipment

Fill in the blank for the selected safety precautions to be followed to avoid accidents and ensure greater client satisfaction.

1. All the electrical appliances you use should be _____ .

2. Read all _____ before using any electrical equipment.

3. _____ all appliances when not in use.

4. _____ all electrical equipment regularly.

5. Keep all wires, plugs, and equipment in good _____ .

6. Use only one plug to each _____ .

7. You and your client should avoid contact with _____ and metal surfaces when using electricity.

8. Do not leave your client unattended while _____ to an electrical device.

9. Keep electrical cords off the _____ and away from people's feet.

10. Do not attempt to _____ around electric outlets while equipment is plugged in.

11. Do not touch two _____ objects at the same time if either is connected to an electric current.

12. Do not step on or place _____ on electrical cords.

13. Do not allow electrical cord to become _____ as it can cause a short circuit.

14. Disconnect appliances by pulling on the _____ , not the cord.

15. Do not attempt to _____ electrical appliances unless you are qualified.

Crossword Puzzle—Electricity

Word	Clue
Electric current	The flow of electricity along a conductor.
Conductor	Any substance that conducts electricity.
Insulator	Or nonconductor is a substance that does not easily transmit electricity.
Direct current	A constant, even-flowing current that travels in one direction only.
Alternating current	A rapid and interrupted current, flowing first in one direction and then in the opposite direction.
Volt	The unit that measures the pressure or force that pushes the flow of electrons forward through a conductor.
Amp	The unit that measures the strength of an electric current.
Milliampere	One-thousandth of an ampere.
Ohm	The unit that measures the resistance of an electric current.
Watt	A measurement of how much electric energy is being used in 1 second.
Fuse	A special device that prevents excessive current from passing through a circuit.

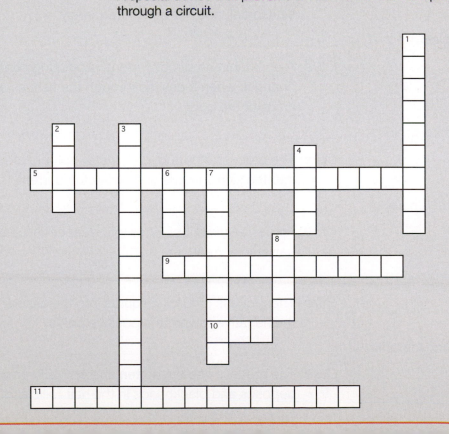

4

Word Scramble—Electricity

Word	Clue
tecdoelre	_ _ _ _ _ _ _ _ _
	Clue: An applicator for directing the electric current from the machine to the client's skin.
alpoytir	_ _ _ _ _ _ _ _
	Clue: Indicates the negative or positive pole of an electric current.
dneao	_ _ _ _ _
	Clue: The positive electrode.
otdehac	_ _ _ _ _ _ _
	Clue: The negative electrode.
aismdloiet	_ _ _ _ _ _ _ _ _ _
	Clue: The four main ones are galvanic, faradic, sinusoidal, and Tesla high frequency.
ngaciavl	_ _ _ _ _ _ _ _
	Clue: A constant and direct current, producing chemical changes when it passes through the tissues and fluids of the body.
ostpohesirnio	_ _ _ _ _ _ _ _ _ _ _ _ _
	Clue: The process of introducing water-soluble products into the skin with the use of electric current.
aporsscthiae	_ _ _ _ _ _ _ _ _ _ _ _
	Clue: Forces acidic substances into deeper tissue using galvanic current.
sipreahosna	_ _ _ _ _ _ _ _ _ _ _
	Clue: The process of forcing liquids into the tissues from the negative toward the positive poles.
oiuttidcsnerans	_ _ _ _ _ _ _ _ _ _ _ _ _ _
	Clue: The process used to soften and emulsify grease deposits and blackheads in the hair follicles.

The Visible Spectrum

Color in the visible spectrum depicted in the diagram using colored pencils, crayons, or water colors.

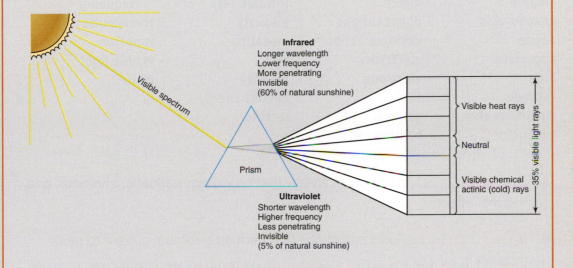

Infrared
Longer wavelength
Lower frequency
More penetrating
Invisible
(60% of natural sunshine)

Visible heat rays

Neutral

Visible chemical
actinic (cold) rays

35% visible light rays

Visible spectrum

Prism

Ultraviolet
Shorter wavelength
Higher frequency
Less penetrating
Invisible
(5% of natural sunshine)

Using the words provided, fill in the blanks below to form a thorough review of Chapter 11: The Basics of Electricity. Words or terms may be used more than once or not at all.

alternating	converter	infrared	tesla high
ampere	direct	infrared rays	frequency
anaphoresis	direct current	kilowatt	therapeutic
anode	desincrustation	modalities	vaporizer
apparatus	electricity	ohm	visible light
blue	electrode	polarity	white
cathode	fuse	radiant energy	
circuit breaker	galvanic	rectifier	
conductor	heating cap	red	

1. _____ is a form of energy that produces magnetic, chemical, and thermal effects.

2. A _____ is a substance that permits electrical current to pass through it.

3. A steamer or _____ produces moist, uniform heat that can be applied to the head or face.

4. A _____ is used to change direct current into alternating current and a _____ is used to change alternating current to direct current.

5. A positive electrode is called a/an _____ and a negative electrode is called a/an _____ .

6. A _____ is a safety device that prevents excessive current from passing through.

7. An amp or _____ is the unit of measurement for the amount of current running through a wire.

8. An _____ is an applicator that directs the electric current from the machine to the client's skin.

ESSENTIAL REVIEW *continued*

9. _____ is the process of forcing liquids into the tissues from the negative toward the positive pole.

10. Artificial light rays are produced by using an electrical _____ called a therapeutic lamp.

11. _____ current is a constant, even-flowing current, traveling in one direction, while _____ current is a rapid and interrupted current, flowing first in one direction then in the opposite.

12. Do not use the negative _____ current on skin with broken capillaries, pustular acne, or on a client with high blood pressure.

13. A switch that automatically interrupts or shuts off an electric circuit at the first indication of overload is a _____ .

14. _____ rays make up 60% of the natural sunlight.

15. The negative or positive state of electric current is _____ .

16. The process used to soften and liquefy grease deposits in the hair follicles and pores is _____ .

17. The _____ light contains few heat rays and has some germicidal and chemical benefits.

18. Another name for electromagnetic radiation is _____ .

19. The _____ current is a thermal or heat-producing current with a high rate of oscillation or vibration.

20. A uniform source of heat can be provided by a _____ .

ESSENTIAL DISCOVERIES AND ACCOMPLISHMENTS

In the space below, jot some notes about what concepts of this chapter were hardest for you to understand or remember. Imagine finding yourself suddenly in the role of "teacher" and consider what you would tell your "students" about these difficult concepts. Share your Essential Discoveries with some of the other students in your class and ask if they are helpful to them. You may want to revise your notes based on good ideas shared by your peers. Under accomplishments, list at least three things you have accomplished since your last entry that relate to your career goals.

Discoveries:

_____

_____

_____

_____

_____

_____

_____

_____

_____

_____

Accomplishments:

_____

_____

_____

_____

_____

PRINCIPLES OF HAIR DESIGN

A Motivating Moment: "*Nothing will be attempted if all possible objections must first be overcome.*"—*Samuel Johnson*

ESSENTIAL OBJECTIVES

After studying this chapter and completing the Essential Companion components, you should be able to:

1. List the five elements of hair design.

2. List the five principles of hair design.

3. Identify different facial shapes.

4. Demonstrate how to design hairstyles to enhance or camouflage facial features.

5. Explain design considerations for men.

ESSENTIAL DESIGN IN HAIRSTYLING

Why is understanding the basic elements of design so important to my success as a cosmetologist?

The answer is as simple as cooking! If you've ever created a masterpiece in the kitchen or even observed a great cook like your mother or grandmother in action, you know that it takes a great deal more than just knowing what the ingredients are. You must know exactly what quantity of each ingredient is needed. You must know at exactly what point each ingredient is added. You need to know things like cooking temperatures and how to use special kitchen tools such as knives or wire whisks. The exact same principles apply in hairstyling. You must attain a thorough knowledge of all the tools and implements required in creating a great design. In addition, you must know the principles of design and also understand how the client's face shape and features impact the chosen design. Once you have gained a solid working knowledge of all these parts, pieces, and principles, you will be able to provide quality services to each and every client.

If there are so many key "ingredients" to hair design, where do I begin?

You must gain an understanding first of the five elements of design which are form, space, line, color, and texture. Then you must experiment with those five elements to create a variety of designs. You must also gain knowledge of the principles of hair design which include proportion, balance, rhythm, emphasis, and harmony, and how each affects the end result. Finally, you must learn about all the client's personal circumstances which will impact the overall design. These include the client's face shape, facial features, head shape, profile, and whether or not the client wears eyeglasses. All of these concepts will be contributing factors as to whether you provide the client with a complimentary and satisfactory hair design.

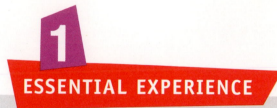

The Elements of Design

Form

Take pictures of the same hairstyle on a client or another student from three different angles. Cut around the perimeter of the hairstyle for each angle and in the area provided below, outline the style in the Essential Companion. Discuss with fellow students how different the silhouette is from different angles. (If a camera is not available for your use, let your creative juices flow. Consider creating a silhouette on the chalkboard in the classroom by adjusting the overhead lighting and using a flashlight or spotlight. Once you've traced three different silhouettes on the chalkboard, copy a smaller version below.)

Space

In order to get a better grasp of what is meant by volume and how the same amount of volume can take on a variety of three-dimensional shapes and styles, try this project. At home in your kitchen, measure out exactly 8 ounces of water and pour it into a round plastic cup. Measure another 8 ounces of water and pour it into a square plastic container. Measure another 8 ounces of water and pour it into a rectangular-shaped plastic container. Place all three containers in the freezer. After they are frozen, remove the frozen masses from their respective containers and compare their shapes. Remember, each ice mold represents the exact same volume of water. *Note:* You can use any size or shape of container for this experiment as long as it is freezer safe.

1 ESSENTIAL EXPERIENCE *continued*

Line

Curly, straight, or curved lines create the form, design, and movement of a hairstyle. Depict the following different lines by cutting pictures out of magazines and paste them in the space provided below. Using a colored pen, emphasize the type of line the style depicts.

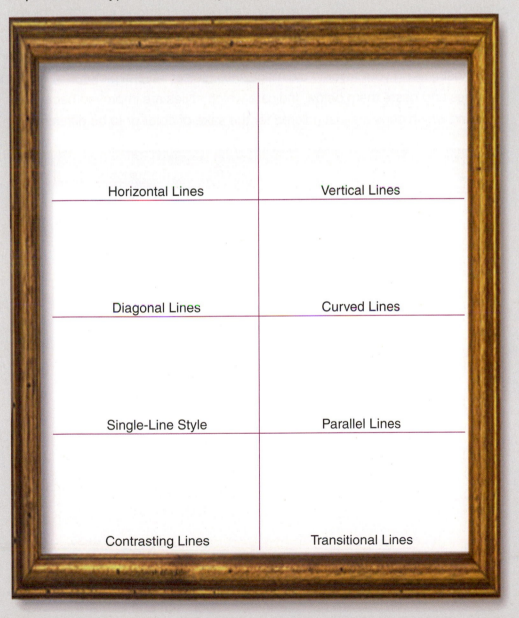

Horizontal Lines	Vertical Lines
Diagonal Lines	Curved Lines
Single-Line Style	Parallel Lines
Contrasting Lines	Transitional Lines

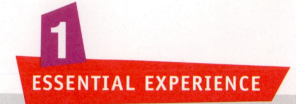

ESSENTIAL EXPERIENCE *continued*

Color

You will learn to use color to bring dimension and finish to the style. Think about a living room that is painted a dull beige with beige carpet and a light brown sofa. It likely appears to be rather dull. Imagine, however, what a difference you could make if you painted one wall a brighter contrasting color or added several throw pillows to the sofa in a variety of textures and colors or added a brightly colored throw rug over the carpet. Imagine the difference any one of those changes would make to the room's overall appearance. The same principle applies to hair color. Again, using your favorite old magazines, select several pictures of different hairstyles and paste them below. Indicate which styles are improved because of color and which ones are just colored for the sake of color or to be different.

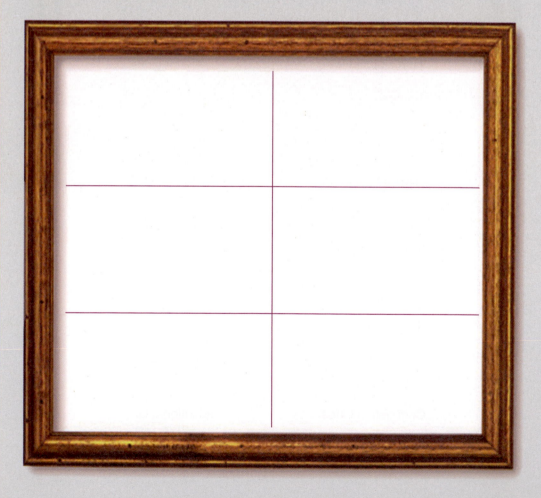

1 ESSENTIAL EXPERIENCE *continued*

Texture

All of us have a natural wave pattern. It may be straight, wavy, curly, or even extremely curly. When aiding our clients in selecting a hairstyle that will be most flattering and easy to maintain, we must take into consideration wave pattern. In this activity, you are being asked to search magazines for pictures that depict various types of wave patterns. Paste them in the spaces provided below and write a brief explanation about the look created by each wave pattern.

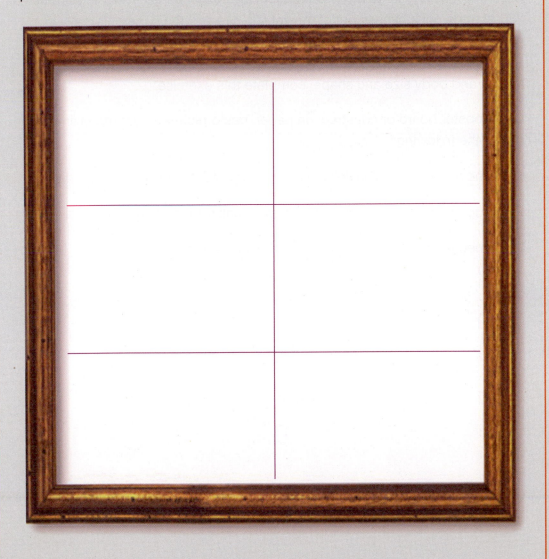

The Principles of Design

Proportion

Proportion deals with the harmonious relationship of the parts of something to each or to the whole. Haven't you ever seen something that is clearly out of proportion with its surroundings? Perhaps you've observed a cute, but extremely tiny, foreign car pull into the parking lot at the mall and then watched as a very large man about 6 feet and 6 inches tall, weighing about 230 pounds hoist himself out of the vehicle. He and the car aren't really in harmony with each other. The same principle applies in hair design. To help you understand the importance of proportion with the face, features, head shape, and body size and shape, complete this exercise.

Using poster board or construction paper, paste pictures from magazines that depict the following:

1. Someone whose hairstyle is much too large for their petite body.

2. Someone whose hairstyle is much too small for their larger body frame.

3. Someone whose hairstyle reflects classic proportions.

2 ESSENTIAL EXPERIENCE *continued*

Balance

By balance we mean that the hairstyle is equal in size or volume around the head. It can be both symmetrical and asymmetrical. Please complete the windowpane activity below.

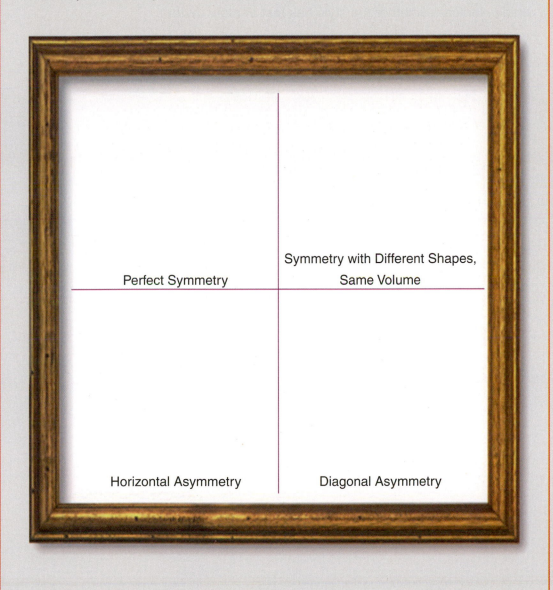

Perfect Symmetry	Symmetry with Different Shapes, Same Volume
Horizontal Asymmetry	Diagonal Asymmetry

2

ESSENTIAL EXPERIENCE *continued*

Rhythm

When you think of someone having great rhythm, you are likely visualizing how they move on a dance floor. Rhythm means the same thing in a hairstyle. It means movement. Cut six different pictures out of magazines and paste them below. Indicate whether the style has fast or slow rhythm.

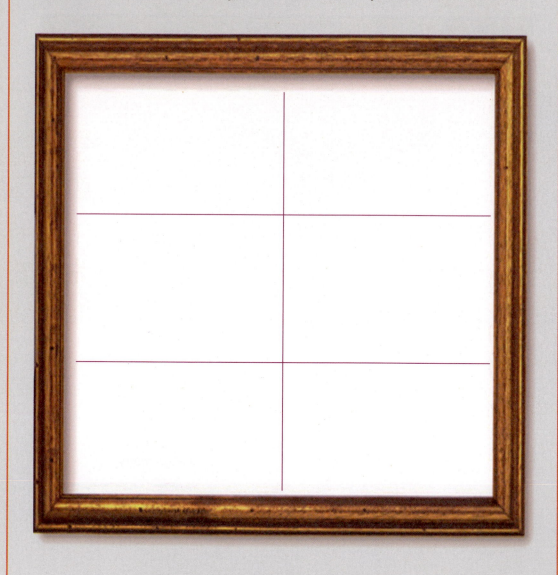

2 ESSENTIAL EXPERIENCE *continued*

Emphasis

Emphasis is the focal point or the point of prominence in the hairstyle. Our eyes tend to see this part of the style first. List a few ideas of how you can add emphasis to a hairstyle.

_____

_____

_____

_____

Harmony

Without harmony, none of the other principles of design will work. Harmony is what holds all the elements of the design together. Think about anyone you've known, a celebrity perhaps, who may have had great color or balance but the harmony just did not happen. List their names here and explain why there was no harmony.

_____

_____

_____

_____

3 ESSENTIAL EXPERIENCE

Windowpane—Facial Types

Windowpaning is the process of transferring key elements, points, or steps in a lesson into visual images that are hand sketched into the squares of "panes" of a matrix. Look through magazines and find pictures that depict the face shapes indicated below. Let your mind think in pictures and sketch the essential concepts printed in each of the following windowpanes.

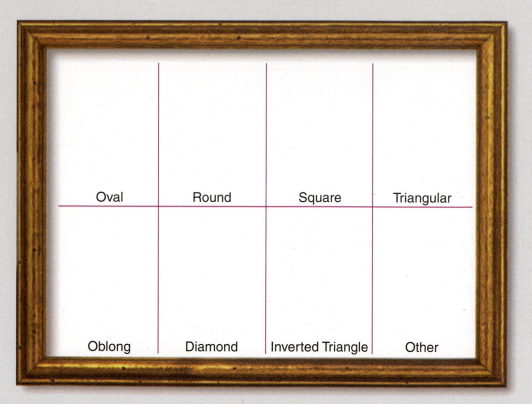

Oval	Round	Square	Triangular
Oblong	Diamond	Inverted Triangle	Other

On a separate sheet of paper, describe the appropriate hairstyle for each of the face shapes listed in the matrix. In the case of magazine pictures, why the hairstyle works or doesn't work.

ESSENTIAL EXPERIENCE

Special Considerations A

Match the following essential terms with their identifying terms or phrases by placing the identifying number next to the appropriate term.

_____ Wide forehead

_____ Close-set eyes

_____ Crooked nose

_____ Square jaw

_____ Long jaw

_____ Convex profile

_____ Large forehead

_____ Prominent nose

_____ Small chin

_____ Large chin

1. Asymmetrical, off-center style is best.

2. Use curved lines at the jaw line.

3. Direct hair forward over the sides of the forehead.

4. A receding forehead and chin.

5. Use bangs with little or no volume.

6. Hair should be full and fall below the jaw.

7. Direct hair back and away from the face at the temples.

8. Bring hair forward at forehead with softness around face.

9. Hair should be longer or shorter than chin.

10. Move hair up and away from face along chin line.

4

Special Considerations B

Match the following essential terms with their identifying terms or phrases by placing the identifying number next to the appropriate term.

_____ Narrow forehead	**1.**	Use straight lines at the jaw line.
_____ Wide-set eyes	**2.**	Direct bangs over the forehead with outward directed volume.
_____ Wide, flat nose	**3.**	Hair should sweep off the face, creating a line from nose to ear.
_____ Round jaw	**4.**	A prominent forehead and chin.
_____ Straight profile	**5.**	Direct hair away from the face at the forehead.
_____ Concave profile	**6.**	Use a higher half bang to create length in the face.
_____ Receding forehead	**7.**	Direct hair forward in the chin area.
_____ Small nose	**8.**	Draw hair away from face, use center part.
_____ Receding chin	**9.**	Ideal profile.

5 ESSENTIAL EXPERIENCE

Crossword Puzzle—Design in Hairstyling

Word	Clue
Asymmetrical	Unequal proportions designed to balance facial features.
Balance	Establishing equal or appropriate proportions to create symmetry.
Concave	Curving inward.
Contrasting	Horizontal and vertical lines that meet at a 90-degree angle.
Convex	Curving outward.
Diagonal	Lines positioned between horizontal and vertical.
Emphasis	Place in a hairstyle where the eye is drawn first.
Form	Outline of the overall hairstyle.
Bang	Triangular section that begins at the apex and ends at the front corners.
Harmony	Orderly and pleasing arrangement of shapes and lines.
Proportion	Harmonious relationship between parts.
Rhythm	Regular, recurrent pattern of movement.
Space	The area the hairstyle occupies.
Symmetrical	Hairstyle design that is similar on both sides of the face.
Transitional	Curved lines used to blend and soften.

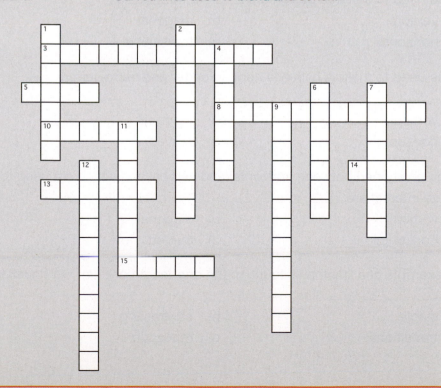

ESSENTIAL REVIEW

Complete the following review of Chapter 12: Principles of Hair Design by circling the correct answer to each question.

1. The outline or silhouette of a hairstyle is known as the _____ .
   a) space   b) line
   c) form   d) design

2. The shape, design, and movement of the hairstyle is created by the _____ .
   a) space   b) lines
   c) form   d) design

3. The area that the hairstyle occupies is called _____ .
   a) space   b) lines
   c) form   d) design

4. Lines that are parallel to the floor are known as _____ .
   a) vertical   b) diagonal
   c) horizontal   d) curved

5. Lines used to soften a design are _____ .
   a) vertical   b) diagonal
   c) horizontal   d) transitional

6. Lines used to make a hairstyle appear longer and narrower are _____ .
   a) vertical   b) diagonal
   c) horizontal   d) curved

7. Lines positioned between horizontal and vertical and which are used to create interest are _____ .
   a) vertical   b) diagonal
   c) horizontal   d) curved

8. An example of a line that is found in the one-length or blunt cut hairstyle is the _____ line.
   a) single   b) contrasting
   c) transitional   d) repeating

ESSENTIAL REVIEW *continued*

9. Lines that meet at a 90-degree angle and create a hard edge are called
   _____ lines.
   a) single
   b) contrasting
   c) transitional
   d) repeating

10. Curved lines used to soften and blend horizontal or vertical lines are
    known as _____ lines.
    a) vertical
    b) contrasting
    c) transitional
    d) repeating

11. Lighter and warmer colors are used to create the illusion of
    _____ .
    a) subtlety
    b) repetition
    c) volume
    d) closeness

12. Dark and cool colors move forward or toward the head and create the
    illusion of less _____ .
    a) volume
    b) height
    c) width
    d) strength

13. When choosing haircolor, it should be compatible with the client's
    _____ .
    a) eye color
    b) skin tone
    c) family's choice
    d) childhood dreams

14. Texture can be natural or created with styling techniques, chemical
    changes, curling irons, or _____ .
    a) client's desire
    b) stylist's desire
    c) hair brushing
    d) hot rollers

15. Curly hair can be permanently straightened with _____ .
    a) curling irons
    b) hair relaxers
    c) pressing irons
    d) crimping irons

16. Curly and extremely curly hair does not reflect much light and could be
    _____ to the touch.
    a) soft
    b) smooth
    c) limp
    d) coarse

17. The five principles of hair design are proportion, balance, rhythm, emphasis, and _____ .
    a) symmetry
    b) asymmetry
    c) harmony
    d) diagonal

18. _____ wave patterns accent the face and are particularly useful when you wish to narrow a round head shape.
    a) rough
    b) busy
    c) smooth
    d) numerous

19. Establishing equal or appropriate proportions to create symmetry is known as _____ .
    a) balance
    b) harmony
    c) rhythm
    d) emphasis

20. The pattern that creates movement in a hairstyle is known as _____ .
    a) balance
    b) harmony
    c) rhythm
    d) emphasis

21. _____ is considered the most important of the principles of hair design.
    a) balance
    b) harmony
    c) rhythm
    d) emphasis

22. The _____ in a hairstyle is the place the eyes see first.
    a) balance
    b) harmony
    c) rhythm
    d) emphasis

23. Generally, the ideal face shape is said to be the _____ shape.
    a) square
    b) round
    c) oval
    d) pear

24. The face is divided into _____ zones.
    a) one
    b) two
    c) three
    d) four

ESSENTIAL REVIEW *continued*

25. The aim of creating the illusion of width in the forehead would be best for the _____ face shape.

  a) round   b) triangular
  c) oblong   d) diamond

26. The aim of reducing the width across the cheekbone line is best for the _____ face shape.

  a) round   b) triangular
  c) oblong   d) diamond

27. The aim of making the face appear shorter and wider is best for the _____ face shape.

  a) round   b) pear
  c) oblong   d) diamond

28. Using a higher half bang to create length in the face would be best for _____ .

  a) a wide forehead   b) close-set eyes
  c) a narrow forehead   d) wide-set eyes

29. Directing the hair forward over the sides of the forehead is best for _____ .

  a) a wide forehead   b) close-set eyes
  c) a narrow forehead   d) wide-set eyes

30. Asymmetrical, off-center styles are best for _____ .

  a) narrow forehead   b) close eyes
  c) long jaw line   d) crooked nose

31. The profile which has a receding forehead and chin is called the _____ profile.

  a) convex   b) concave
  c) straight   d) curved

32. The profile which has a prominent forehead and chin is called the _____ profile.

  a) convex   b) concave
  c) straight   d) curved

ESSENTIAL REVIEW   *continued*

33. Bangs with little or no volume should be used for a _____ .
a) receding forehead
b) large forehead
c) low forehead
d) small forehead

34. A part that helps develop height on top and make thin hair appear fuller is the _____ part.
a) center
b) side
c) diagonal
d) zigzag

35. The _____ part should be used to create width or height in a hairstyle.
a) triangular
b) diagonal
c) side
d) zigzag

36. The _____ part is used to create a dramatic effect.
a) triangular
b) diagonal
c) side
d) zigzag

37. The _____ part is considered to be the basic parting for the bang section.
a) triangular
b) diagonal
c) side
d) zigzag

38. The _____ part is used to direct hair across the top of the head.
a) triangular
b) diagonal
c) side
d) center

39. The _____ part is considered to be the classic part and is usually used for an oval face, but can be used to create the illusion of oval for a round or wide face.
a) curved
b) side
c) center
d) diagonal

40. The _____ part is used for a receding hairline or high forehead.
a) curved
b) side
c) center
d) diagonal

ESSENTIAL DISCOVERIES AND ACCOMPLISHMENTS

In the space below, jot some notes about what concepts of this chapter were hardest for you to understand or remember. Imagine finding yourself suddenly in the role of "teacher" and consider what you would tell your "students" about these difficult concepts. Share your Essential Discoveries with some of the other students in your class and ask if they are helpful to them. You may want to revise your notes based on good ideas shared by your peers. Under Accomplishments, list at least three things you have accomplished since your last entry that relate to your career goals.

Discoveries:

_____

_____

_____

_____

_____

_____

_____

_____

_____

Accomplishments:

_____

_____

_____

_____

_____

SHAMPOOING, RINSING, AND CONDITIONING

A Motivating Moment: "Do not go where the path may lead; go instead where there is no path and leave a trail."—Ralph Waldo Emerson

ESSENTIAL OBJECTIVES

After studying this chapter and completing the Essential Companion components, you should be able to:

1. Explain pH and its importance in shampoo selection.

2. Explain the role of surfactants in shampoo.

3. Discuss the uses and benefits of various types of shampoos and conditioners.

4. Perform proper scalp manipulations as part of a shampoo service.

5. Demonstrate proper shampooing and conditioning procedures.

ESSENTIAL SHAMPOOING AND CONDITIONING

Why are shampooing and conditioning so important to my training when they seem to be such insignificant services?

Just because you have been shampooing and conditioning your own hair for a number of years does not mean that you have appropriate knowledge to deliver a professional shampoo and conditioning service to your clients. It is necessary to understand that the procedure and various products that you have used at home are likely not professional products and may not be client oriented. In fact, it is not uncommon for people to choose their shampoo or conditioning treatment based on its fragrance or because talented marketing managers suggest it is beneficial for their hair.

Your ability to provide a thorough and pleasing shampoo is essential. It is generally the first service you provide a client and allows you to begin building a positive client relationship. More importantly, the shampoo service is the most repeated service you provide your clients. In most cases, a thorough shampoo will precede a haircut, a style, a color treatment, and any chemical reformation. You can be sure that how well you perform the shampoo service will greatly impact the client's perception of how well you will perform other services they desire. And remember, when you give a good shampoo with a relaxing scalp massage, you lay the groundwork for selling the client many more services both today and in the future!

ESSENTIAL CONCEPTS

What do I need to know about shampooing, rinsing, and conditioning in order to provide a quality service?

It may help you to understand some history about cleansing the hair. The word shampoo is derived from the Hindu word *champna* which means to press, knead, or shampoo. History tells us that humankind has found many ways to cleanse the body in order to prevent disease. They used natural ingredients to accomplish this, including soapwort which is a plant that produces a lather in water. Near the middle of the 20th century, however, scientists created chemical ingredients to replace the natural ones. Chemists became aware of the pH (potential hydrogen) level of hair and recognized that products should be created that would maintain the natural pH of the hair.

You will also need to know how important proper brushing is before the shampoo service. You will then need to practice and master the shampoo procedure. Once you have accomplished that, you will want to achieve a keen understanding of the chemistry of shampoos, rinses, and conditioning treatments and the effects that those chemicals will have on the hair. You, as a professional cosmetologist, actually become the client's hair "physician." Therefore, your knowledge of the effects of various products on the hair will be critical in your role as a professional consultant who prescribes treatments for the hair.

1

ESSENTIAL EXPERIENCE

Find a partner and conduct a research project on the various shampoo products used in your school. You may want to expand your project by researching the shampoo products used at home by both partners. Use the following chart to list each type of shampoo, the type of hair they are created for, and the ingredients found in each. After you have collected the data, make a determination regarding any common ingredients in the products. Finally, obtain some litmus paper and test each product to determine the pH level (level of acidity and alkalinity) of each.

Product Name	Recommended for Which Hair Type	Ingredients	pH Level

After identifying the common ingredients, write a brief explanation of why you believe these ingredients are used in so many shampoo products.

_____

_____

_____

_____

2

ESSENTIAL EXPERIENCE

Using the pH scale provided below, label the pH levels of the shampoos you researched in Essential Experience 1.

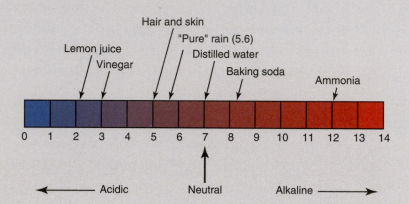

3 ESSENTIAL EXPERIENCE

Collect hair swatches for various types of hair including normal, color-treated, relaxed, and permed. Shampoo the swatches at least five times with one available shampoo product, using a different shampoo for each swatch. Report the effects of the shampoo on each swatch. Then divide each swatch in half and condition one half. Report on the effects of each shampoo on each swatch. Report on the results after half the swatch has been reconditioned. Tape the swatches into the box provided.

Swatch Type	Shampoo Used	Results	Conditioned Swatch	Results
Normal				
Color Treated				
Relaxed				
Permed				

Make recommendations for the ideal shampoo for each hair type and explain why others are not appropriate.

_____

_____

_____

13

4 ESSENTIAL EXPERIENCE

Arrange to have both soft and hard water available for use for this experiment. Using the different water types and a professional shampoo product, compare the product's lathering ability, cleansing ability, and the appearance of the hair afterward. Record your results below.

_____

_____

_____

_____

_____

_____

_____

_____

5

ESSENTIAL EXPERIENCE

Number the following shampoo scalp manipulations in the order they should occur.

_____ Allow the client's head to relax and work around the hairline with your thumbs in a rotary movement.

_____ Continue in this manner to the back of the head, shifting your fingers back one inch.

_____ Drop you fingers down one inch and repeat the process until the right side of the head is covered.

_____ Begin at the front hairline and work in a back-and-forth movement until the top of the head is reached.

_____ Repeat these movements until the scalp has been thoroughly massaged.

_____ Lift the client's head, with your left hand controlling the movement of the head. With your right hand, start at the top of the right ear and, using the same movement, work to the back of the head.

_____ Remove excess shampoo and lather by squeezing the hair.

_____ Beginning at the left ear, repeat steps 3 and 4.

6 ESSENTIAL EXPERIENCE

Crossword Puzzle—Shampooing, Rinsing, and Conditioning

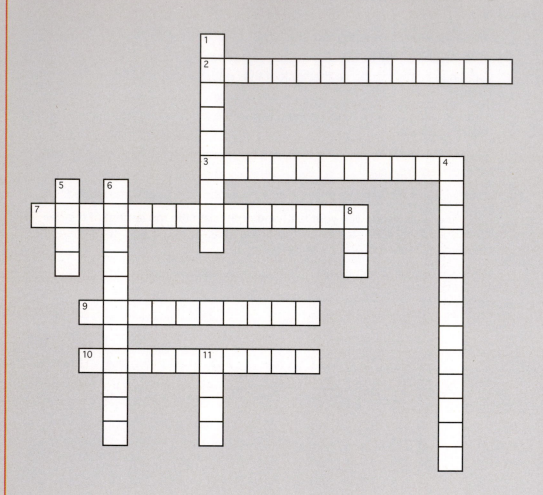

Across

2. Having a balanced pH
3. Moisturizes, restores, and protects hair
7. Shampoo created by combining the surfactant base with basic dyes
9. Detergent
10. Attract oil

Down

1. Shampoo that washes away excess oiliness
4. Another name for conditioner
5. Rain water or chemically treated water
6. Adds moisture to hair
8. Shampoo that cleanses without soap and water
11. Water containing minerals that lessen the ability to lather

ESSENTIAL RUBRICS

Rubrics are used in education for organizing and interpreting data gathered from observations of student performance. It is a clearly developed scoring document used to differentiate between levels of development in a specific skill performance or behavior. A rubric is provided in this study guide as a self-assessment tool to aid you in your behavior development.

Rate your performance according to the following scale:

(1) Development Opportunity: There is little or no evidence of competency;
Assistance is needed; Performance includes multiple errors.

(2) Fundamental: There is beginning evidence of competency;
Task is completed alone; Performance includes few errors.

(3) Competent: There is detailed and consistent evidence of competency;
Task is completed alone; Performance includes rare errors.

(4) Strength: There is detailed evidence of highly creative, inventive, mature presence of competency.

Space is provided for comments to assist you in improving your performance and achieving a higher rating.

SCALP MANIPULATION AND TREATMENT PROCEDURE

Performance Assessed	1	2	3	4	Improvement Plan
Gathered supplies and implements					
Pre-service sanitation and set up completed					
Washed and Sanitized hands					
Properly draped client and performed scalp analysis					
Explained scalp and hair condition and recommended treatment					
Performed relaxing movement					
Performed sliding movement					
Performed sliding and rotating movement					
Performed forehead movement					
Performed rotary scalp movement					
Performed hairline movement					
Performed front and back scalp movements					
Performed ear-to-ear movement					
Performed back movement					
Performed Shoulder movement					
Performed spine movement					
Post-service cleanup					

ESSENTIAL RUBRICS—CONT'D

SHAMPOOING PROCEDURE

Performance Assessed	1	2	3	4	Improvement Plan
Gathered implements and supplies					
Pre-service sanitation and set up completed					
Washed and sanitized hands					
Properly draped client and removed objects from hair					
Examined scalp and brushed hair thoroughly					
Re-draped client; placed drape outside shampoo chair					
Adjusted volume and temperature of water					
Saturated hair and applied shampoo					
Manipulated scalp					
Rinsed hair thoroughly; repeated shampoo/rinse					
Removed excess water and applied conditioner					
Rinse thoroughly					
Towel dry and detangle hair					
Performed post-service cleanup; proceeded to next service					

ESSENTIAL REVIEW

Using the following words, fill in the blanks to form a thorough review of Chapter 13: Shampooing, Rinsing, and Conditioning. (Please note that the appropriate pages in the textbook are referenced but should not be referred to until you have completed the questions based on your own knowledge.) Words or terms may be used more than once or not at all.

0 to 6.9	astringent lotions	humectants	tangles
blood	4.5 to 5.5	acid	protein
condition	brittle	7.1 to 14	citric acid
H_2O_2	polymers	chemical service	H_2O
medicated	hard	dry	ingredients
scales	natural	hydrogen	powder
soft	shampooing	oily	skin
volume	stimulating	shampoos	temperature

1. An important preliminary first step for a variety of hair services is _____ .

2. To be effective, a shampoo must remove all dirt, oils, cosmetics, and _____ debris without adversely affecting either the scalp or hair.

3. _____ hair should be shampooed more often than other types.

4. Hair can usually be characterized as oily, _____ , normal, or chemically treated.

5. Rain water or water that has been chemically treated is known as _____ water.

6. _____ water contains certain minerals that lessen the ability of the shampoo to lather readily.

7. _____ bristles are recommended for hair brushing.

8. Select the shampoo according to the _____ of the client's hair.

9. A high pH shampoo can leave the hair dry and _____ .

10. You should not brush the hair prior to giving a _____ .

ESSENTIAL REVIEW   *continued*

11. Brushing stimulates the _____ circulation to the scalp and helps remove dust, dirt, and hair spray buildup from the hair.

12. You should never use a comb to loosen _____ from the scalp.

13. The inner side of your wrist is used to test the water _____ .

14. Biotin and protein are conditioning agents that restore moisture and elasticity, strengthen the hair shaft, and add _____ .

15. _____ account for the highest dollar expenditure in hair care products.

16. The key to determining which shampoo will leave the hair shiny and manageable is the _____ list.

17. The amount of _____ in a solution determines whether it is more alkaline or more acid.

18. Shampoos that are more acid will fall in the range of _____ on the pH scale.

19. Shampoos that are more alkaline will fall in the range of _____ on the pH scale.

20. An acid-balanced shampoo will fall in the range of _____ on the pH scale.

21. _____ shampoos contain special chemicals that are effective in reducing excessive dandruff.

22. A _____ shampoo is usually given when the client's health does not permit a regular shampoo.

23. Most conditioners contain silicone along with moisture-binding _____ that absorb moisture or promote the retention of moisture.

24. Penetrating conditioners that are left on the hair for 10 to 20 minutes restore _____ and moisture.

25. Scalp _____ remove oil accumulation from the scalp and are used after a scalp treatment.

ESSENTIAL DISCOVERIES AND ACCOMPLISHMENTS

In the space below, jot some notes about what concepts of this chapter were hardest for you to understand or remember. Imagine finding yourself suddenly in the role of "teacher" and consider what you would tell your "students" about these difficult concepts. Share your Essential Discoveries with some of the other students in your class and ask if they are helpful to them. You may want to revise your notes based on good ideas shared by your peers. Under Accomplishments, list at least three things you have accomplished since your last entry that relate to your career goals.

Discoveries:

_____

_____

_____

_____

_____

_____

_____

_____

_____

Accomplishments:

_____

_____

_____

_____

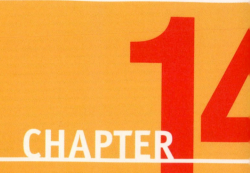

HAIRCUTTING

A Motivating Moment: "Courage is the first of human virtues because it makes all others possible." —Aristotle

ESSENTIAL OBJECTIVES

After studying this chapter and completing the Essential Companion components, you should be able to:

1. Identify reference points on the head form and understand their role in haircutting.

2. Define angles, elevations, and guidelines.

3. List the factors involved in a successful client consultation.

4. Demonstrate the safe and proper use of the various tools of haircutting.

5. Demonstrate mastery of the four basic haircuts.

6. Demonstrate mastery of other haircutting techniques.

ESSENTIAL HAIRCUTTING

I really want to specialize in hair design, so why is it so important for me to master the art of haircutting?

Haircutting is a technique that requires many hours of practice and a vivid imagination. It is an extremely important skill that must be mastered because the cut serves as the basis for every hairstyle. It may not be done as frequently as a shampoo or style, but it is certainly completed more frequently than chemical services. If you want to ensure that the style you provide your client is the most attractive and will look good even when he or she styles his or her own hair, you must deliver a quality haircut. The way to accomplish that is with frequent practice, repetitive exercises, timed procedures, and a strong desire to become an accomplished haircutter.

ESSENTIAL CONCEPTS

What are the most important techniques and procedures I should learn to become a good haircutter?

Haircutting is actually more than just reducing length and bulk from the hair. It begins with using quality tools, and there are many to aid you in achieving a dynamic haircut. You will want practice techniques with shears, razors, clippers, thinning shears, and all the ancillary tools such as combs and brushes. You will want to work with all these tools until you have complete control and can handle them with ease. You will need to become familiar with all the terms used in haircutting. It is important to remember that terminology in our industry constantly changes. Don't let yourself get sidetracked because one instructor or one book calls a specific cut one thing and another calls it something else. It's the end result that matters, not what the technique, procedure, or style is named.

Your instructor will take you through steps of sectioning for various types of cuts. You will find that proper sectioning is extremely important, especially until you have learned to manage and control larger amounts of hair. You will learn all about angles and elevations and how to combine them to create a wide variety of hairstyles. It is highly recommended that you style every haircut you complete while learning. This allows you to see the results of your efforts. If, for example, you are unable to achieve the desired style after the cut, it may be because you haven't yet mastered that particular haircut. Just remember that no one performs a perfect haircut the first time. It takes practice and commitment—so don't give up.

1

ESSENTIAL EXPERIENCE

Identify the Tools

Using the photos found below, please label each tool using the following terms (some terms may be used more than once).

Back	Barber comb	Blade
Finger grip	Finger tang	Finger rest
Handle	Head	Heel
Pivot	Pivot screw	Point
Shoulder	Still blade	Styling comb
Tang	Thinning shears	Edge
Wide-tooth comb	Haircutting shears	Moving blade
Shank	Tail comb	

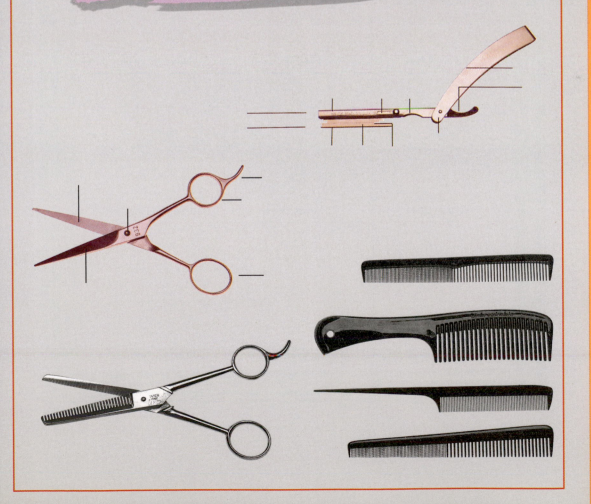

2 ESSENTIAL EXPERIENCE

Windowpane

Windowpaning is the process of transferring key elements, points, or steps in a lesson into visual images that are hand sketched into the squares or "panes" of a matrix. Let your mind think in pictures and sketch the essential concepts printed in each of the following windowpanes. Don't be concerned with your artistic ability. Use lines and stick figures to depict each concept.

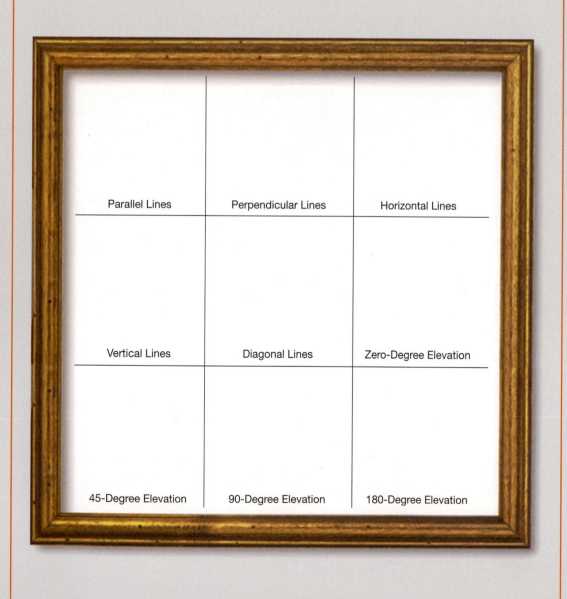

Parallel Lines	Perpendicular Lines	Horizontal Lines
Vertical Lines	Diagonal Lines	Zero-Degree Elevation
45-Degree Elevation	90-Degree Elevation	180-Degree Elevation

3

ESSENTIAL EXPERIENCE

Terms—A

Match the essential terms with their identifying terms or phrases.

_____ Beveling	**1.**	Lines that are between horizontal and vertical.
_____ Haircutting shears	**2.**	Outer line.
_____ Thinning shears	**3.**	Used to remove superfluous hair and to create clean lines around ears and neckline.
_____ Razor	**4.**	Used to create very short tapers quickly.
_____ Clippers	**5.**	Usually used to cut a blunt straight line; can be used to thin hair by slithering.
_____ Edgers	**6.**	Lines that are parallel to the floor; used in low elevation haircuts.
_____ Angle	**7.**	Space between two lines that intersect.
_____ Perimeter	**8.**	Used to remove bulk from the hair.
_____ Horizontal lines	**9.**	Used to cut hair with a softer edge than shears.
_____ Diagonal lines	**10.**	Cutting the ends of the hair at a slight taper.

3 ESSENTIAL EXPERIENCE *continued*

Terms—B

Match the essential terms with their identifying terms or phrases.

_____ Blunt cut	**1.**	Cutting with the points of the shears to create texture in the hair ends.
_____ Elevation	**2.**	This shape has a stacked area around the exterior and is cut at low to medium elevations.
_____ Graduated	**3.**	Graduated effect achieved by cutting the hair with elevation or over-direction.
_____ Guideline	**4.**	Section of hair that determines the length the hair will be cut.
_____ Layering	**5.**	Level at which a blunt cut falls; where the ends of the hair hang together.
_____ Notching or point cutting	**6.**	Line dividing the hair to create subsections.
_____ Parting	**7.**	How tightly the hair is pulled before cutting.
_____ Sections	**8.**	Lines that are perpendicular to the floor.
_____ Tension	**9.**	Cutting the hair straight across the strand. All hair hangs to one level, forming a weight line.
_____ Weight line	**10.**	Divisions of the hair made before cutting.
_____ Vertical lines	**11.**	Angle at which the hair is held away from the head for cutting.

4

ESSENTIAL EXPERIENCE

Windowpaning is the process of transferring key elements, points, or steps in a lesson into visual images that are hand sketched into the squares or "panes" of a matrix. Let your mind think in pictures and sketch the essential concepts printed in each of the following windowpanes. Don't be concerned with your artistic ability. Use lines and stick figures to depict the concepts requested.

Haircutting Concepts

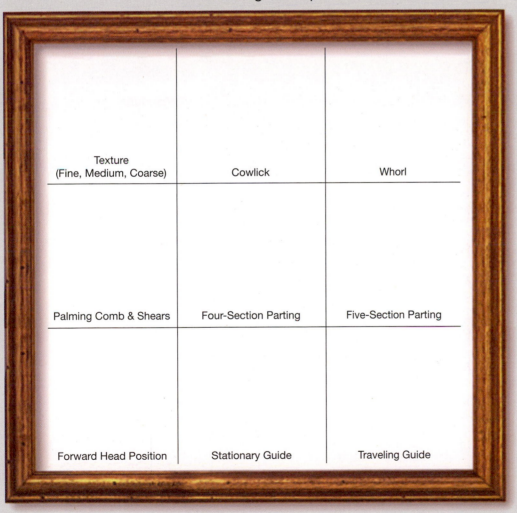

Texture (Fine, Medium, Coarse)	Cowlick	Whorl
Palming Comb & Shears	Four-Section Parting	Five-Section Parting
Forward Head Position	Stationary Guide	Traveling Guide

5

ESSENTIAL EXPERIENCE

As a professional stylist you will have numerous clients who bring in photographs because they want to achieve the same or similar look. Therefore, learning how to evaluate a style and determine how it was achieved will be of great benefit to you. With that in mind, look through various magazines and select three particular cuts that appeal to you. Paste them on the chart below in the left column. In the right column, diagram and/or explain the techniques, angles, and elevations you would use to create this particular haircut and style.

Paste Picture Here	Procedure
Paste Picture Here	Procedure
Paste Picture Here	Procedure

6

Word Scramble

Scramble	Correct Word
ntlub uct	_ _ _ _ _ _ _ _ *Clue:* Cut straight across
adterudga	_ _ _ _ _ _ _ _ _ *Clue:* A wedge or stack
nergif	_ _ _ _ _ _ *Clue:* Triangular section that begins at apex and ends at front corners
egrynial	_ _ _ _ _ _ _ _ *Clue:* Cutting the hair with elevation or overdirection
iseontcs	_ _ _ _ _ _ _ *Clue:* Divisions in hair before cutting
ladnioag	_ _ _ _ _ _ _ _ *Clue:* Between horizontal and vertical
lenaigvrt	_ _ _ _ _ _ _ _ _ *Clue:* Moving
liavctre	_ _ _ _ _ _ _ _ *Clue:* Perpendicular to the floor
diew hotot	_ _ _ _ _ _ _ _ _ _ *Clue:* Comb used to create softer edge when cutting with shears
sderge	_ _ _ _ _ _ *Clue:* Remove superfluous hair
utsenoicsb	_ _ _ _ _ _ _ _ _ _ *Clue:* Partings
hrlwo	_ _ _ _ _ *Clue:* Requires extra length
zroar	_ _ _ _ _ *Clue:* Cuts hair with softer edge

7

ESSENTIAL EXPERIENCE

Word Search—Haircutting

After determining the correct words from the clues provided, locate the words in the word search puzzle.

Word	Clue
_____	Used for close tapers
_____	Holding the shears at an angle other than 90 degrees to the hair strand
_____	A cut that is short on the bottom and long on the top
_____	Cheaters
_____	Found in the hairline or the interior of the hair
_____	Slithering
_____	The angle at which the hair is held away from the head
_____	Section of hair that determines the length
_____	90-degree haircut
_____	Lines that are parallel to the floor

```
B A R B E R C O M B M G L Q T B
I N S X W E C H D Q V M S W L I
H K E D L F B C H F M W N E D G
M Q I D R Q U P I G Y O N W P T
Y E A W I A B S F R I D Q C F B
N M Q S S U U Q Q T E E M N U G
O R N X P X G G A D J C H R J N
I I X T C S Q V H Q V A O J X I
T Q H B C Y E T S T L T X I O T
A H D W P L H S P L G V W T K A
V M C E E T R X I G C N P D K L
E G L H G A N K Y V B I E X Y I
L V G E W E N J U H V R L L Y F
E I A F D J J I I S H S E Q C F
H H O R I Z O N T A L Z F F O E
B E V E L E D C U T W B X I C C
```

8 ESSENTIAL EXPERIENCE

In your owns words, explain the purpose of the following procedures.

Checking a Haircut
One possible response follows:

_____

_____

_____

_____

Slide Cutting
One possible response follows:

_____

_____

_____

_____

Shears-Over-Comb Technique
One possible response follows:

_____

_____

_____

_____

9
ESSENTIAL EXPERIENCE

Word Search

After determining the correct words from the clues provided, locate the words in the word search puzzle.

Word	Clue
_____	Traveling
_____	Also known as pointing
_____	Lines that never meet in space
_____	Subsections
_____	A popular barbering technique
_____	Used to cut a blunt straight line across the hair
_____	Stable
_____	How tightly the hair is pulled when cutting
_____	Removing bulk without removing length
_____	Level at which the blunt cut falls

```
P Y Q R X X M X G O M K F T S N Z I
M A G S U R G M X G A Y A T O D H Q
X E R K Q Y E T S U Y O A I I A S U
S W U T B M H A Q B K T S H W V Z N
C F A S I M F E S T I N B V I C Z V
G F Q Y R N O A E O E C K P O P J H
I R H V S P G C N T G Y P G R L K C
S K Q E A G N A R P S C J R A V S F
D Z B N N E R G E E A D E O W V I G
Z F T W P Y N G Q N V R M N U A M L
Q N S D G I N S H W I O A N Q X D J
M P B U H I U K S S Q L S L M Y M R
M O I C N Z U N T S Q V T R L K R O
H D T D U X D B P D P M H A E C Z
E O I D L W A T Q T S E A H G E L A
N H R I G I H C F J D H Z L H I H R
T G C Z A B J A X Y U J X F G E E S
M O V I N G K W E J L J J Q H J T O W
```

ESSENTIAL RUBRICS

Rubrics are used in education for organizing and interpreting data gathered from observations of student performance. It is a clearly developed scoring document used to differentiate between levels of development in a specific skill performance or behavior. A rubric is provided in this study guide as a self-assessment tool to aid you in your behavior development.

Rate your performance according to the following scale:

(1) Development Opportunity: There is little or no evidence of competency; Assistance is needed; Performance includes multiple errors.

(2) Fundamental: There is beginning evidence of competency; Task is completed alone; Performance includes few errors.

(3) Competent: There is detailed and consistent evidence of competency; Task is completed alone; Performance includes rare errors.

(4) Strength: There is detailed evidence of highly creative, inventive, mature presence of competency.

Space is provided for comments to assist you in improving your performance and achieving a higher rating.

BLUNT HAIRCUT PROCEDURE

Performance Assessed	1	2	3	4	Improvement Plan
Pre-service sanitation and set up completed					
Washed and sanitized hands					
Performed client consultation					
Properly draped, shampooed, towel-dried hair					
Detangled hair; combed away from face					
Performed center and ear to ear partings					
Positioned head upright and created 1st subsection at nape					
Combed subsection, positioned fingers and shears parallel to parting					
Created guideline by cutting straight across					
Repeat on other side of head					
Cut next sections from side to side up to crown					
At crown, combed hair into natural fall					
Perform horizontal parting at side hairline to back section					
Combed subsection, positioned fingers and shears parallel to parting					
Cut horizontal line to back guide					
Continued up side till complete					
Repeated cutting procedure on opposite side					

14

ESSENTIAL RUBRICS—CONT'D

BLUNT HAIRCUT PROCEDURE—cont'd

Performance Assessed	1	2	3	4	Improvement Plan
Cross-checked haircut using vertical sections					
Post-service cleanup and appointment scheduling completed					

GRADUATED HAIRCUT PROCEDURE

Performance Assessed	1	2	3	4	Improvement Plan
Pre-service sanitation and set up completed					
Washed and sanitized hands					
Performed client consultation					
Properly draped, shampooed, towel-dried hair					
Detangled hair; combed away from face					
Parted hair into 6 sections					
Established guideline at center of nape section					
Used a horizontal cutting line parallel to fingers; cut right and left sides of nape					
Worked upward in left back section cutting to guide					
Established vertical section at center part; extended to nape guide					
Combed subsection at 45° angle to scalp; held fingers at a 90° angle to strand, cut					
Cut entire horizontal section in same manner; blended each section					
Continued cutting back sections with hair becoming longer at apex					
Cut crown at 90° angle while cutting; blend back and crown					
Established left side guide and cut					
Established right side guide and cut					
Established hairline guide and cut					
Cut from nape to side					

ESSENTIAL RUBRICS—CONT'D

GRADUATED HAIRCUT PROCEDURE—cont'd

Performance Assessed	1	2	3	4	Improvement Plan
Established horizontal guide on side and cut					
Established vertical section at ear and cut					
Continued cutting left side, blended side and top					
Cut right side, blended side and top					
Created fringe guide, cut left and right side of fringe blending at center and sides					
Cut top section to blend with crown and fringe until cut was complete					
Post-service cleanup and appointment scheduling completed					

UNIFORM LAYERS HAIRCUT PROCEDURE

Performance Assessed	1	2	3	4	Improvement Plan
Pre-service sanitation and set up completed					
Washed and sanitized hands					
Performed client consultation					
Properly draped, shampooed, towel-dried hair					
Detangled hair; combed away from face					
Established two partings from hairline to nape about ½" apart					
Parted out first section at crown and cut					
Continued cutting guideline to front hairline					
Continued cutting guideline from crown to nape					
For control, parted hair from apex to back of ear; worked through back first					
Wedge-shaped, vertical partings were used from apex to nape					
Followed traveling guide, cut right side beginning at crown to back of ear					
Repeated procedure on left side					

14

ESSENTIAL RUBRICS—CONT'D

UNIFORM LAYERS HAIRCUT PROCEDURE—cont'd

Performance Assessed	1	2	3	4	Improvement Plan
Cross-checked back area					
Clipped sides out of the way; Sectioned off top area					
Cut top area using vertical partings; blended with guide					
Cross-checked top using horizontal partings					
Cut right side from back of ear to face; repeated on left					
Cross-checked side sections					
Combed hair down					
Post-service cleanup and appointment scheduling completed					

LONG LAYERS HAIRCUT PROCEDURE

Performance Assessed	1	2	3	4	Improvement Plan
Pre-service sanitation and set up completed					
Washed and sanitized hands					
Performed client consultation					
Properly draped, shampooed, towel-dried hair					
Detangled hair; combed away from face					
Parted hair into five cutting sections					
Began at top crown with 2" subsection across head; combed hair straight up and cut straight across					
Worked to front of top section by taking 2"subsections; cut to same length					
On left side, used 2" horizontal subsections combed to match previously cut hair in top section					
Continued working down side till hair no longer reached guide					
Repeated procedure on right side					
At top of left rear section, used 2" horizontal subsections; combed hair straight up from hear form					

ESSENTIAL RUBRICS—CONT'D

LONG LAYERS HAIRCUT PROCEDURE—cont'd

Performance Assessed	1	2	3	4	Improvement Plan
Continued from top to bottom until hair no longer reaches guideline					
Repeated procedure on left side					
Post-service cleanup and appointment scheduling completed					

MEN'S BASIC CLIPPER CUT PROCEDURE

Performance Assessed	1	2	3	4	Improvement Plan
Pre-service sanitation and set up completed					
Washed and sanitized hands					
Performed client consultation					
Properly draped, shampooed, towel-dried hair					
Detangled hair; combed away from face					
Established a horseshoe parting 2" below apex that began and ended at hairline					
Started at nape; placed comb against scalp from 0 to 45°; cut over comb					
Repeated cutting step up back of head					
Cross-cut horizontally from side to side					
Cut sides of back from ear to ear using the clipper over comb technique					
Blended lengths over curve of head by cross-cutting					
Using small number attachment, cut sideburns to the parietal ridge					
Measured from eyebrow to natural hairline					
Cut narrow guideline at crown end of horseshoe parting					
Began at crown, cut top to initial crown guideline					
Moved toward forehead, pulled hair back toward guideline to increase length					

14

MEN'S BASIC CLIPPER CUT PROCEDURE—cont'd

Performance Assessed	1	2	3	4	Improvement Plan
Using clipper and attachment, shortened and shaped hair around ears					
Finished cut ensuring head and length were in harmony					
Used clipper or trimmer to blend or outline perimeter					
Post-service cleanup and appointment scheduling completed					

ESSENTIAL REVIEW

Complete the following review of Chapter 14: Haircutting, by circling the correct answer to each question.

1. Cutting all the hair to one length is a/an _____ cut.
   a) elevation
   b) blunt
   c) graduated
   d) beveled

2. A cut that has a stacked area around the exterior and is cut at low to medium elevations is a/an _____ cut.
   a) elevation
   b) blunt
   c) graduated
   d) beveled

3. Cutting with the points of the shears to create texture is known as _____ .
   a) layering
   b) undercutting
   c) elevation
   d) notching

4. Subdivisions of a section, used for control when cutting are known as _____ .
   a) subsections
   b) guides
   c) sections
   d) tension

5. If the hair is cut partially wet and partially dry, the results will be _____ .
   a) even
   b) perfect
   c) uneven
   d) curly

6. The tools also known as trimmers that are used to clean necklines and around the ears are _____ .
   a) clippers
   b) edgers
   c) razor
   d) shears

7. A tool used to cut blunt straight lines is called the _____ .
   a) clippers
   b) edgers
   c) razor
   d) shears

8. The tool used to cut hair with a softer edge is known as the
   _____ .

   a) clippers   b) edgers

   c) razor   d) shears

9. The comb used for close tapers in the nape and sides is the
   _____ comb.

   a) styling   b) barber

   c) wide-tooth   d) tail

10. The comb used mainly to detangle the hair is the _____ comb.

    a) styling   b) barber

    c) wide-tooth   d) tail

11. _____ points are points on the head that mark where the surface
    of the head changes or the behavior of the hair changes, such as the ears,
    jawline, occipital bone, or apex.

    a) parietal   b) crown

    c) elevation   d) reference

12. _____ lines are parallel to the floor.

    a) horizontal   b) perpendicular

    c) diagonal   d) vertical lines

13. Lines that are perpendicular to the floor are _____ lines.

    a) parallel   b) perpendicular

    c) diagonal   d) vertical

14. A haircutting technique that is measured in degrees is _____ .

    a) carving   b) elevation

    c) clipper-over-comb   d) traveling

15. Lines that are used for blending and stacking are _____ lines.

    a) parallel   b) perpendicular

    c) diagonal   d) vertical

16. A stable guide that does not move is also known as a _____
    guide.

    a) moving   b) traveling

    c) stationary   d) mobile

ESSENTIAL REVIEW *continued*

17. When the hair is cut at 90 degrees and higher, the result is a
_____ haircut.
a) blunt   b) layered
c) graduated   d) blended

18. A 180-degree haircut is also known as a _____ .
a) low elevation cut   b) combined elevation cut
c) long layered haircut   d) blended elevation cut

19. A zero-degree haircut is also known as a _____ elevation.
a) low   b) high
c) reverse   d) blended

20. A barbering technique that has become popular with cosmetologists is
the _____ -over-comb method.
a) clipper   b) razor
c) trimmer   d) shears

21. A/an _____ is a thin continuous mark used as a guide.
a) angle   b) line
c) elevation   d) section

22. Gliding the fingers and shears along the edge of the hair to remove length
is called _____ cutting.
a) point   b) slide
c) notching   d) razor

23. The process of thinning with scissors is known as _____ .
a) effilating   b) shaving
c) sliding   d) trimming

24. _____ guides are used mostly in blunt (one-length) haircuts
or when using overdirection to create a length or weight increase in a
haircut.
a) traveling   b) movable
c) stationary   d) portable

25. _____ is used mostly in graduated and layered haircuts, and
in those situations where a length increase in the design is desired.
a) effilating   b) trimming
c) elevating   d) overdirection

14

In the space below, jot some notes about what concepts of this chapter were hardest for you to understand or remember. Imagine finding yourself suddenly in the role of "teacher" and consider what you would tell your "students" about these difficult concepts. Share your Essential Discoveries with some of the other students in your class and ask if they are helpful to them. You may want to revise your notes based on good ideas shared by your peers. Under Accomplishments, list at least three things you have accomplished since your last entry that relate to your career goals.

Discoveries:

_____

_____

_____

_____

_____

_____

_____

_____

_____

_____

_____

Accomplishments:

_____

_____

_____

_____

_____

HAIRSTYLING

A Motivating Moment: "If you are looking for a big opportunity, find a big problem."—Unknown

ESSENTIAL OBJECTIVES

After studying this chapter and completing the Essential Companion components, you should be able to:

1. Demonstrate (a) finger waving, (b) pin curls, (c) roller setting, and (d) hair wrapping.

2. Demonstrate various blow-dry styling techniques.

3. Demonstrate three basic techniques of styling long hair.

4. Demonstrate the proper use of thermal irons.

5. Demonstrate various thermal iron manipulations and explain how they are used.

6. Describe the three types of hair pressing.

7. Demonstrate the procedures involved in soft pressing and hard pressing.

ESSENTIAL WET HAIRSTYLING

What roles will wet hairstyling, thermal hairstyling, and hair pressing play in my success as a cosmetologist?

Hairstyles, like fashions, are cyclical. Just as you've seen the bell-bottom pants of the late 1960s come into fashion again, hairstyles, such as those that were popular in the 1920s, surface from time to time in our society. History has shown that all societies have cut and arranged hair to modify its natural state. The pages of our history books depict great diversity from decade to decade. They show the blond wigs of Roman matrons, the gray wigs of English barristers, and the black wigs of Japanese geisha. We also see the sleek, waved look worn by the flappers in the 1920s and the trend toward informality and individualism in the 21st century.

Recent surveys of today's modern salons indicate that the new stylists joining their teams must be skilled in many styling techniques, including thermal styling and curling. History shows us that thermal or heat techniques have been used for centuries to create certain looks. The heat from the sun was used to speed up the processing of hair lighteners, permanent waves, and hair color. Hair was wrapped around reeds and sticks and sun-dried for certain looks. Fortunately, the tools and implements have improved drastically since those primitive times.

Marcel Grateau developed the thermal iron technique in 1875, which is still called marcel waving today. The use of blow-drying and curling irons became really popular in the late 1960s with the first "bob" cut and has become increasingly popular into the 21st century as more women have entered the business world and time is so critical. These techniques are used for what are called "quick services" in the salon. However, the same care must be taken with these techniques as with wet hairstyling.

Hair pressing is both a popular and profitable service that is used in many of today's professional establishments. Overly curly hair comes in many colors, textures, and ethnicity. We have all heard the expression, "the grass looks greener on the other side of the fence." Accordingly, we human beings always seem to want something that we don't have. If we have straight hair, we want

15

it to be curly; therefore we seek out chemical texture services to add curl to our hair. If we have naturally curly hair, we want it to be straight; therefore we seek out either pressing or chemical services to remove the curl. All those desires contribute to your success as a professional cosmetologist.

Once you become a professional cosmetologist, you will hold your license or certification for many years to come, hopefully over several decades. You must be prepared to address your client's desires and needs regardless of the prevailing styles of the times. Therefore, it is essential that you learn the basics of hairstyling in order to be proficient in providing the client's desired style.

What are the most important elements in hairstyling that I need to know?

Hairstyling is an art form; hair is the medium and you are the artist. Hairstyling results from a detailed set of principles, elements, tools, and implements. You will need to learn to master the use of the tools and implements used in hairstyling as well as how to properly prepare the hair for the styling service. You will become familiar with a variety of styling aids which do just that—aid you in creating the desired look or style. You will learn that finger waving is the art of shaping and directing the hair into alternate parallel waves with well-defined ridges using the fingers, combs, waving lotion, and hairpins, or clips.

You will learn how the concept of waves evolves into the concept of curls, including pin curls and roller curls. There are a variety of techniques for creating pin curls and roller sets that will allow you to work your magic as an artist in your medium of hair. You will also master several brushing and combing procedures that will allow you to give the finished look to the style you have designed.

In addition, thermal styling is the art of drying, waving, and curling hair by means of heat, using special manipulative techniques. It includes drying and styling the hair, curling or waving the hair, and straightening the hair. Each piece of equipment used in thermal styling is designed for a specific styling technique. The essential techniques that you must master are the use of the blow-dryer and the curling iron. You will need to know how each piece of equipment functions and how to create a variety of looks with each.

You will need to also learn about the three types of hair pressing techniques, the soft press, the medium press, and the hard press. It is essential that you understand which type of press is used on which type of hair. Of course, you will also need to master each of the techniques. Learning about special problems with pressing and fine tuning all the safety measures that must be followed will also contribute to your success.

ESSENTIAL EXPERIENCE

1

Mind Map of Wet Hairstyling

Mind mapping simple creates a free-flowing outline of material or information with the central or key point being located in the center. The key point of this mind map is wet hairstyling. Diagram the different tools, implements, and elements or categories of wet hairstyling. Use terms, pictures, and symbols as desired. Using color will increase the mind's retention and memory of the material. Keep your mind open and uncluttered and don't worry about where a line or word should go as the organization of the map will usually take care of itself.

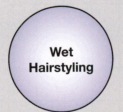

Wet
Hairstyling

2 ESSENTIAL EXPERIENCE

Windowpane—Pin Curls

Windowpaning is the process of transferring key elements, points, or steps in a lesson into visual images that are hand sketched into the squares or "panes" of a matrix. Let your mind think in pictures and sketch the essential concepts printed in each of the following windowpanes. Don't be concerned with your artistic ability. Use lines and stick figures to depict the concepts indicated.

Parts of a Pin Curl	No-Stem Curl	No-Stem Curl Opened
Half-Stem Curl	Full-Stem Curl	Proper Anchoring of Pin Curl
Clockwise Curls and Counterclockwise Curls	Stand-Up Curl	Barrel Curl

Follow-up Activity: Perform each of the following curls or movements on a mannequin for a grade from your instructor.

____ No-Stem Curl ____ Half-Stem Curl ____ Full-Stem Curl

____ Clockwise Curl ____ Stand-Up Curl ____ Barrel Curl

Pin Curl Shaping and Bases

Match the following essential terms with their identifying phrase or definition.

_____ Circular

_____ Oblong

_____ Shaping

_____ Ridge curl

_____ Spiral curl

_____ Carved curls

_____ Closed

_____ Rectangular

_____ Triangular

_____ Arc base

_____ Square base

_____ Ribboning

1. Pin curls sliced from a shaping and formed without lifting the hair from the head.

2. Pie-shaped with the open end smaller than the closed end. In a wave pattern, the direction is alternated.

3. Recommended along the front or facial hairline to avoid breaks or splits in the finished style.

4. Remains the same width throughout the shaping.

5. Used for even construction suitable for curly hairstyles without much volume or lift.

6. Also known as the half-moon or c-shaped base.

7. Recommended at front hairline for a smooth upsweep effect.

8. Section of hair molded in a circular motion.

9. Pin curls that produce waves that get base smaller in size toward the end.

10. Pin curls placed behind or below a ridge to form a wave.

11. Forcing the strand through the comb while applying pressure with the thumb on the back of the comb to create tension.

12. Method of curling hair by winding strand around the rod.

4 ESSENTIAL EXPERIENCE

Windowpane—Roller Placement

Windowpaning is the process of transferring key elements, points, or steps in a lesson into visual images that are hand sketched into the squares or "panes" of a matrix. Let your mind think in pictures and sketch the essential concepts printed in each of the following windowpanes. Don't be concerned with your artistic ability. Use lines and stick figures to depict the concepts indicated.

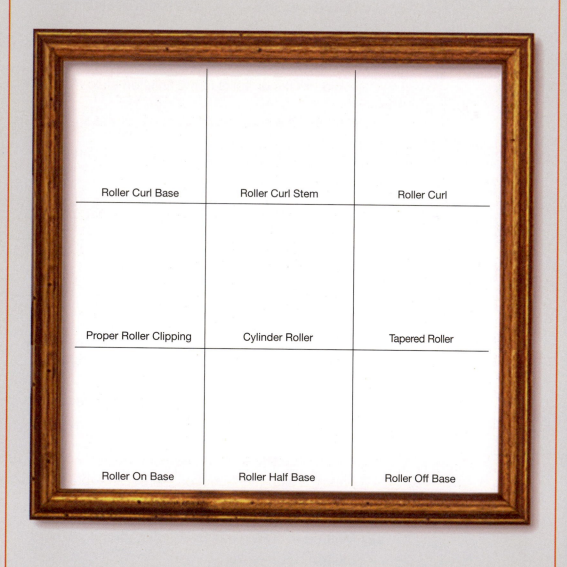

Roller Curl Base	Roller Curl Stem	Roller Curl
Proper Roller Clipping	Cylinder Roller	Tapered Roller
Roller On Base	Roller Half Base	Roller Off Base

ESSENTIAL EXPERIENCE

Word Search

After identifying the appropriate word from the clues listed below, locate the word in the following word search puzzle.

Word	Clue
_____	Also called ruffing.
_____	Pin curls with large openings; fastened to head in a standing position on a rectangular base.
_____	Pin curls sliced from a shaping and formed without lifting the hair from the head.
_____	Nozzle attachment that directs the air flow.
_____	Blow-dryer attachment that causes air to flow more softly.
_____	Technique of passing a hot curling iron through the hair before performing a hard press.
_____	Produces a strong curl with full volume.
_____	Removes 100% of the curl by applying the pressing comb twice on each side of the hair.
_____	Curl placed directly on its base.
_____	Forces hair between the thumb and back of comb to create tension.
_____	Pin curls placed immediately behind or below a ridge to form a wave.
_____	Round, solid prong of a thermal iron.
_____	Part of thermal irons in which rod rests when irons are closed.
_____	Two rows of ridge curls, usually on the side of head.
_____	Method of curling the hair by winding a strand around the rod.
_____	Also called cascade curls.
_____	Section of pin curl between the base and first arc.
_____	Hairstyle arranged up and off the shoulders.
_____	Type of gel that makes hair pliable for finger waving.

5

ESSENTIAL EXPERIENCE *continued*

```
S  L  R  U  C  L  E  R  R  A  B  S  T  G  M
L  R  U  C  L  A  R  I  P  S  B  G  N  N  K
R  E  S  N  O  I  T  O  L  G  N  I  V  A  W
U  S  L  D  S  M  T  R  G  I  H  U  Q  K  Q
C  U  R  W  O  I  O  O  N  S  S  U  M  X
P  F  U  S  M  U  O  O  U  N  S  W  S  M  B
U  F  C  B  L  P  B  R  S  H  E  L  L  E  U
-  I  D  M  D  B  B  L  Q  W  R  A  F  T  R
D  D  E  H  I  -  J  D  E  U  P  D  O  S  H
N  O  V  R  K  V  X  Y  C  P  D  F  E  -  T
A  X  R  C  O  N  C  E  N  T  R  A  T  O  R
T  L  A  E  P  H  G  N  I  C  A  E  R  N  N
S  B  C  J  J  D  F  O  K  J  H  D  S  H  B
Z  R  S  K  I  P  W  A  V  E  S  Z  H  S  Q
I  T  J  R  E  S  A  B  -  L  L  U  F  S  T
```

6 ESSENTIAL EXPERIENCE

Iron Manipulations

Using a cold thermal iron, a mannequin, and other required implements, practice the textbook exercises for manipulating thermal irons.

Exercise 1: Since it is important to develop a smooth rotating movement, practice turning the irons while opening and closing them at regular intervals. Practice rotating the irons downward toward you and upward away from you.

Exercise 2: Practice releasing the hair by opening and closing the irons in a quick, clicking movement.

Exercise 3: Practice guiding the hair strand into the center of the curl as you rotate the irons. This exercise will ensure that the end of the strand is firmly in the center of the curl.

Exercise 4: Practice removing the curl from the irons by drawing the comb to the left and the rod to the right. Use the comb to protect the scalp from burns.

After completing the exercises, please explain any difficulties you may have had with the exercises in the space below. Discuss these difficulties with your instructor.

_____

_____

_____

_____

_____

_____

_____

_____

7 ESSENTIAL EXPERIENCE

Safety Precautions

In the space provided, please explain why the following safety precautions are necessary in the use of thermal waving and curling.

1. Irons should not be overheated.

2. The temperature of the irons must be tested before applying to hair.

3. Irons should be handled carefully.

4. Irons should be placed in a safe place to cool.

5. Handles should not be placed too close to the heater when heating the irons.

6. Irons should be properly balanced when placed in the heater.

7. Celluloid combs or metal combs cannot be used.

8. Combs with broken teeth must not be used.

9. Comb must be placed between scalp and thermal iron when curling or waving.

10. Hair ends must not be allowed to protrude over the irons.

11. Thermal irons are generally not used on chemically straightened hair.

12. A first aid kit must be readily available.

8 ESSENTIAL EXPERIENCE

Thermal Curling Preparation

Please list the four general steps used in preparing for an electric or stove-heated thermal curling iron procedure. Bear in mind that these methods may be changed by your instructor.

1. _____
   _____
   _____
   _____

2. _____
   _____
   _____
   _____

3. _____
   _____
   _____
   _____

4. _____
   _____
   _____
   _____

5. _____
   _____
   _____
   _____

9 ESSENTIAL EXPERIENCE

Windowpaning—Thermal Curling

Windowpaning is the process of transferring key elements, points, or steps in a lesson into visual images that are hand sketched into the squares or "panes" of a matrix. Let your mind think in pictures, and sketch the essential concepts printed in each of the following windowpanes. Don't be concerned with your artistic ability. Use lines and stick figures to depict the concepts requested.

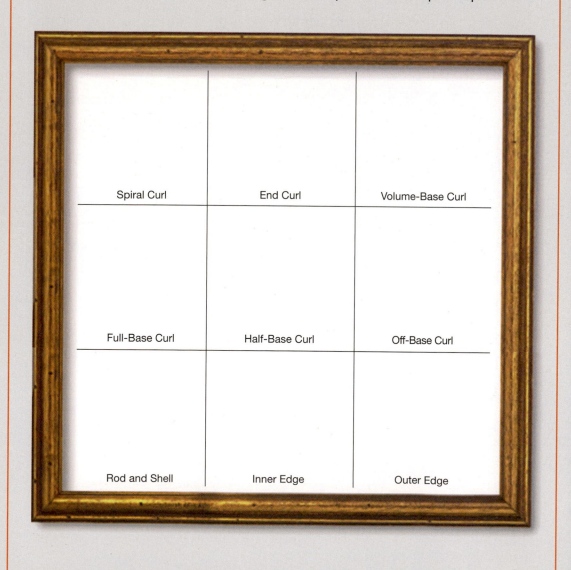

Spiral Curl	End Curl	Volume-Base Curl
Full-Base Curl	Half-Base Curl	Off-Base Curl
Rod and Shell	Inner Edge	Outer Edge

ESSENTIAL EXPERIENCE

Thermal Waving With Conventional Thermal Irons

List below the equipment, implements, and materials used in thermal waving with a conventional thermal (marcel) iron.

_____

_____

In your own words, list the basic procedural steps which can be used to create a style with a conventional thermal (marcel) iron for a left-going wave.

1. _____
_____
_____
_____
_____

2. _____
_____
_____
_____

3. _____
_____
_____
_____

4. _____
_____
_____
_____
_____

10

5. _____
_____
_____
_____
_____
_____

6. _____
_____
_____
_____
_____

7. _____
_____
_____
_____
_____

8. _____
_____
_____
_____
_____

9. _____
_____
_____
_____
_____
_____

10

ESSENTIAL EXPERIENCE *continued*

10. _____

    _____

    _____

    _____

    _____

11. _____

    _____

    _____

    _____

12. _____

    _____

    _____

    _____

    _____

11

Types of Hair Pressing

In your own words in the space provided, explain what is meant by each type of pressing technique and how each is accomplished.

Soft Press: _____

_____

_____

Medium Press: _____

_____

_____

Hard Press: _____

_____

_____

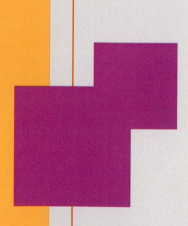

12

ESSENTIAL EXPERIENCE

Product Knowledge

Research a variety of pressing oils or creams available in your school and found at local supply stores. Use the chart below to track your findings.

Product Name	Key Ingredients	Purpose	Benefits	Directions for Use

13

Hair and Scalp Analysis

List the eight points that should be thoroughly covered in the hair and scalp analysis before proceeding with a hair pressing service.

1. _____
2. _____
3. _____
4. _____
5. _____
6. _____
7. _____
8. _____

List at least five reminders and hints on soft pressing.

1. _____
   _____
2. _____
   _____
3. _____
   _____
4. _____
   _____
5. _____
   _____
6. _____
   _____
7. _____
   _____

14

ESSENTIAL EXPERIENCE

Jeopardy

As in the game Jeopardy, write questions that would be correctly answered as follows:

Hair Pressing for $100.

1. To temporarily straighten overly curly or unruly hair.

_____

_____

2. A series of conditioning treatments.

_____

_____

3. Soft, medium, hard.

_____

_____

Hair Pressing for $200.

1. Double press.

_____

_____

2. Breakage.

_____

_____

3. Medium hair.

_____

_____

14
ESSENTIAL EXPERIENCE *continued*

Hair Pressing for $300.

1. Scalp abrasions, contagious scalp condition, scalp injury, chemically treated hair.

_____

_____

2. Wiry, curly hair.

_____

_____

3. Regular and electric.

_____

_____

Hair Pressing for $400.

1. Carbon.

_____

_____

2. Apply less pressure to the hair near the ends.

_____

_____

Rubrics are used in education for organizing and interpreting data gathered from observations of student performance. It is a clearly developed scoring document used to differentiate between levels of development in a specific skill performance or behavior. A rubric is provided in this study guide as a self-assessment tool to aid you in your behavior development.

Rate your performance according to the following scale:

(1) Development Opportunity: There is little or no evidence of competency; Assistance is needed; Performance includes multiple errors.

(2) Fundamental: There is beginning evidence of competency; Task is completed alone; Performance includes few errors.

(3) Competent: There is detailed and consistent evidence of competency; Task is completed alone; Performance includes rare errors.

(4) Strength: There is detailed evidence of highly creative, inventive, mature presence of competency.

Space is provided for comments to assist you in improving your performance and achieving a higher rating.

WET SET WITH ROLLERS PROCEDURE

Performance Assessed	1	2	3	4	Improvement Plan
Pre-service sanitation and set up completed					
Washed and sanitized hands					
Performed client consultation and properly draped client					
Combed hair in direction of setting pattern					
Applied setting lotion if needed					
Started at front hairline, parted off section the length and width of roller					
Select base according to desired volume; combed hair section till smooth					
Placed smoothly wrapped rollers					
Clipped rollers securely to scalp hair					
Placed client under hair dryer					
Removed rollers and styled hair as desired					
Post-service cleanup and appointment scheduling completed					

HORIZONTAL FINGER WAVING PROCEDURE

Performance Assessed	1	2	3	4	Improvement Plan
Pre-service sanitation and set up completed					
Washed and sanitized hands					
Performed client consultation					
Properly draped, shampooed, towel-dried hair					

15

ESSENTIAL RUBRICS—CONT'D

HORIZONTAL FINGER WAVING PROCEDURE—cont'd

Performance Assessed	1	2	3	4	Improvement Plan
Detangled hair, combed hair with natural growth pattern					
Applied waving lotion					
Began on right side and placed index finger in center of shape and molded circular movement					
Formed and completed first ridge					
Reversed direction and formed next ridge					
Continued fingerwaving until right side was complete					
Ensured waves and ridges were blended without splits or breaks					
Placed net over waves and client under the dryer					
Completed style as desired					
Post-service cleanup and appointment scheduling completed					

CARVED OR SCULPTURED CURLS PROCEDURE

Performance Assessed	1	2	3	4	Improvement Plan
Pre-service sanitation and set up completed					
Performed client consultation					
Washed and sanitized hands					
Properly draped, shampooed, towel-dried hair					
Applied styling product					
Formed first shaping					
Started at open end, sliced and ribboned strand					
Wound curl and secured with clip					
Clips entered circle parallel to stem in center of circle					
Used cascade or barrel curls as style dictates					
Dried hair and styled as desired					
Post-service cleanup and appointment scheduling completed					

15

ESSENTIAL RUBRICS—CONT'D

BLOW-DRY BLUNT OR LONG LAYERED HAIRCUT PROCEDURE

Performance Assessed	1	2	3	4	Improvement Plan
Pre-service sanitation and set up completed					
Performed client consultation					
Washed and sanitized hands					
Properly draped, shampooed, towel dried hair					
Detangled hair, removed excess moisture, applied styling product					
Prepared blow dryer					
Established horizontal partings across nape					
Placed brush; dried base, mid-strand, then ends; cooled after drying					
Using same technique, worked up to crown					
Used round brush if more volume was desired					
Used same technique on sides, crown and top					
Used under or over bevel with brush as desired					
Finished fringe as desired					
Completed style as desired					
Post-service cleanup and appointment scheduling completed					

BLOW DRY SHORT LAYERED, CURLY HAIR PROCEDURE

Performance Assessed	1	2	3	4	Improvement Plan
Pre-service sanitation and set up completed					
Performed client consultation					
Washed and sanitized hands					
Properly draped, shampooed, towel-dried hair					
Applied styling product					
Sectioned hair according to desired curl size					

15

ESSENTIAL RUBRICS—CONT'D

BLOW DRY SHORT LAYERED, CURLY HAIR PROCEDURE
—cont'd

Performance Assessed	1	2	3	4	Improvement Plan
Used round brush and dried either full base or half base					
Over-directed base if maximum lift was desired					
Used cooling button to strengthen curl formation					
Properly released brush by unwinding					
Completed style as desired; used finishing spray as needed					
Post-service cleanup and appointment scheduling completed					

THERMAL CURLING SHORT HAIR PROCEDURE

Performance Assessed	1	2	3	4	Improvement Plan
Pre-service sanitation and set up completed					
Performed client consultation					
Washed and sanitized hands					
Properly draped, shampooed, towel-dried hair					
Sectioned and parted bases to match desired curl size					
Combed hair smooth and straight out from scalp					
Heated irons to desired temperature					
Picked up strands and combed smoothly					
With groove on top, inserted irons about 1" from scalp and held to form base					
Held ends of hair using medium tension and turned irons downward					
Opened and closed irons rapidly to prevent binding					
Guided ends of strand into center of curl as irons were rotated.					
Continued until finished curls was achieved.					
Post-service cleanup and appointment scheduling completed					

ESSENTIAL RUBRICS—CONT'D

CHIGNON STYLE PROCEDURE

Performance Assessed	1	2	3	4	Improvement Plan
Pre-service sanitation and set up completed					
Performed client consultation					
Washed and sanitized hands					
Draped, shampooed, and dried hair					
Parted hair on desired side and brushed into a low ponytail at nape					
Secured ponytail with elastics; kept hair smooth					
Wrapped small section around elastics to cover					
Back-brushed ponytail from underneath and gently smoothed					
Rolled hair under to form chignon; secured with bobby pins					
Finished with strong finishing spray					
Added ornamentation as desired					
Post-service cleanup and appointment scheduling completed					

CLASSIC FRENCH TWIST PROCEDURE

Performance Assessed	1	2	3	4	Improvement Plan
Pre-service sanitation and set up completed					
Performed client consultation					
Washed and sanitized hands					
Performed wet set or used electric rollers or thermal irons					
Sectioned crown area and two side sections					
Back-combed back section					
Gently smoothed hair to one side of head and secured hair with bobby pins					

15

CLASSIC FRENCH TWIST PROCEDURE—cont'd

Performance Assessed	1	2	3	4	Improvement Plan
Brushed hair from left side over center line and twisted from center of nape					
Tucked ends into fold creating a funnel shape and secured seam with pins					
Tucked all ends into top of twist and pinned					
Lightly back-brushed side sections and smoothed					
Twisted, looped, and pinned side sections.					
Styled fringe area as desired					
Sprayed with firm-holding finishing spray					
Post-service cleanup and appointment scheduling completed					

ESSENTIAL REVIEW

Using the following words, fill in the blanks below to form a thorough review of Chapter 15: Hairstyling. Words or terms may be used more than once or not at all.

anchored	decrease	no	rollers
arc	direction	oblong	ruffing
back combing	drying	off	shallow
barrel	finger waving	on	silicone
base	finishing	pinching	smooth
c-shaped	flattering	pin curls	square
carved	full-stem	pins	stand-up
circle	gel	pliable	stem
circular	hairpins	pomade	tapered
clockwise	horizontal	pushing	tension
counterclockwise	indentation	rectangular	unpigmented
curls	invisible	ribboning	vertical
cylinder	karaya	ridge	visible

1. A stylist's goal is to create a style that is both _____ and easy to manage.

2. Open center curls produce even _____ waves and uniform curls.

3. In _____ finger waving, ridges are parallel around the head.

4. One complete turn around the roller will create a _____ curl.

5. The art of shaping and directing the hair into alternate parallel waves and designs is _____ .

6. The three parts of a pin curl are _____ , _____ , and _____ .

7. The finished result will be determined by the _____ you place the stem of the curl.

8. Curls formed in the opposite direction of the movement of the hands of a clock are known as _____ .

ESSENTIAL REVIEW *continued*

9. Forcing a strand of hair through a comb while applying pressure with the thumb on the back of the comb to create tension is called _____ .

10. _____ are used to create many of the same effects as stand-up pin curls.

11. Two and a half turns around the roller will create _____ .

12. Curls formed in the same direction as the movement of the hands of a clock are known as _____ .

13. The most commonly shaped base you will use is the _____ base.

14. Cascade or _____ curls are used to create height.

15. For the least volume, the roller sits _____ base.

16. Tools and implements required in wet hairstyling include rollers, clips, combs, brushes, and _____ .

17. Waving lotion makes the hair _____ and keeps it in place during the finger waving procedure.

18. A _____ curl allows for the greatest mobility.

19. Waving lotion is applied to one side of the head at a time to prevent _____ .

20. _____ provide the bases for patterns, lines, waves, curls, and rolls that you can use to create hairstyles.

21. Closed center curls produce waves that _____ in size.

22. Do not try to increase the height or depth of a ridge by _____ or _____ with fingers.

23. Waving lotion is made from _____ gum.

ESSENTIAL REVIEW *continued*

24. A loose roller will lose its _____ and result in a weak set.

25. Secure finger waves with _____ or clippies if needed.

26. In _____ finger waving, ridges run up and down the head.

27. Back brushing is also known as _____ .

28. _____ is a firm-bodied and usually clear or transparent product that comes in a tube or bottle and has a strong hold.

29. To ensure that the curl holds firmly, it should be _____ correctly.

30. Pin curls recommended at the side front hairline for smooth upsweep effect are _____ bases.

31. Pin curls sliced from a shaping without lifting hair from the head are referred to as _____ curls.

32. For full volume, the roller sits _____ base.

33. Large stand-up pin curls on a rectangular base with large center openings are known as _____ curls.

34. Teasing, ratting, matting, or French lacing are also known as _____ .

35. _____ or wax adds considerable weight to the hair by causing strands to join together.

36. A _____ stem curl produces a tight, firm, long-lasting curl.

37. _____ adds gloss and sheen to the hair while creating textural definition.

38. A _____ curl is a wave behind the ridge.

39. The most widely used hairstyling product is hair spray or _____ spray.

15

continued

Please complete the following multiple choice by circling the correct answer.

40. When blow-drying, determine the size of the brush to be used by the desired style and _____ of the hair.
a) elasticity
b) texture
c) length
d) porosity

41. The styling parts of the thermal iron are comprised of the rod and the _____ .
a) groove
b) handle
c) shell
d) clamp

42. The temperature of the heated thermal iron is tested on _____ .
a) wax paper
b) hair strand
c) damp cloth
d) tissue paper

43. Curling with two loops is also known as _____ curling.
a) end
b) spiral
c) figure-eight
d) half-base

44. The technique of waving and curling the hair known as marcel waving is also called _____ .
a) blow-drying
b) thermal waving
c) heat rolling
d) finger waving

45. Combs for thermal curling should be made of _____ .
a) celluloid
b) hard rubber
c) plastic
d) soft rubber

46. To give a finished appearance to hair ends, use _____ curls.
a) figure-eight
b) loop
c) figure-six
d) end

47. For successful blow-dry styling, the air should be directed from the scalp to the _____ .
a) floor
b) ceiling
c) face
d) ends

ESSENTIAL REVIEW *continued*

48. When the blow-dry style is complete, the scalp must be _____ .
a) oily
b) moist
c) damp
d) dry

49. Overheated irons are often ruined because the metal loses its

_____ .

a) color
b) balance
c) temper
d) strength

50. Electric vaporizing irons should not be used on pressed hair because they cause the hair to _____ .
a) break
b) dry
c) straighten
d) revert

51. _____ hair withstands less heat in a thermal styling service than normal hair.
a) lightened
b) healthy
c) coarse
d) curly

52. A conventional thermal iron is _____ heated.
a) electric
b) self
c) coal
d) stove

53. _____ hair, as a rule, can tolerate more heat than fine hair.
a) red
b) coarse
c) oily
d) short

54. Spiral curls are hanging curls that are suitable for _____ hairstyles.
a) short
b) clipped
c) long
d) straight

55. Until dexterity is achieved and ease of manipulation is mastered, it is best to practice with _____ irons.
a) cold
b) hot
c) warm
d) rigid

56. How long does a hair press last?

a) a week   b) till the next haircut

c) overnight   d) till the next shampoo

57. The types of hair pressing are soft, medium, and _____ .

a) light   b) hard

c) extreme   d) heavy

58. The temperature of the pressing comb and the amount of pressure used are adjusted based on the _____ of the hair.

a) texture   b) length

c) style   d) cleanliness

59. Which type of hair requires the most pressure and heat?

a) fine   b) medium

c) normal   d) wiry

60. Which type of hair requires less pressure and heat than any other type?

a) fine   b) medium

c) coarse   d) wiry

61. When pressing gray hair, use moderate heat and _____ .

a) more pressing oil   b) moderate pressure

c) less pressure   d) a larger pressing comb

62. Applying a heated comb twice on each side of the hair is known as _____ .

a) regular press   b) hard press

c) soft press   d) comb press

63. Test the temperature of a pressing comb on _____ .

a) inner wrist   b) terry cloth towel

c) light paper   d) dark paper

64. Burnt hair strands _____ .

a) need extra pressing oil   b) occur in hard presses

c) cannot be straightened   d) cannot be conditioned

ESSENTIAL REVIEW *continued*

65. Using excess heat on gray, tinted, or lightened hair may _____ the hair.
    a) discolor
    b) highlight
    c) strengthen
    d) curl

66. Failure to correct dry and brittle hair can result in hair _____ during hair pressing.
    a) curling
    b) discoloration
    c) strengthening
    d) breakage

67. Hair pressing treatments between shampoos are called _____ .
    a) re-presses
    b) re-do's
    c) touch-ups
    d) soft press

68. Before performing a hair press, the hair should be sectioned into _____ main sections.
    a) 3
    b) 4
    c) 5
    d) 9

69. Carbon may be removed from the pressing comb by rubbing with a _____ .
    a) wet towel
    b) pressing oil
    c) strong alcohol
    d) fine steel wool

70. In a hair pressing procedure, the actual pressing or straightening of the hair is accomplished with the comb's _____ .
    a) back rod
    b) wide teeth
    c) warm handle
    d) narrow tail

71. After cleaning the comb's surface, immerse the comb in a hot _____ solution for about 1 hour to give the metal a smooth and shiny appearance.
    a) 70% alcohol
    b) baking soda
    c) soapy water
    d) clear ammonia

72. When pressing _____ hair, use a moderately heated pressing comb applied with light pressure.
    a) coarse
    b) thick
    c) long
    d) unpigmented

73. Pressing combs should be constructed of good-quality stainless steel or
_____ .

a) zinc   b) rubber

c) brass   d) plastic

74. In pressing coarse hair, more heat is required because it has the greatest
_____ .

a) elasticity   b) length

c) porosity   d) diameter

75. Handles of pressing combs are usually made of _____ .

a) wood   b) steel

c) carbon   d) brass

ESSENTIAL DISCOVERIES AND ACCOMPLISHMENTS

In the space below, jot some notes about what concepts of this chapter were hardest for you to understand or remember. Imagine finding yourself suddenly in the role of "teacher" and consider what you would tell your "students" about these difficult concepts. Share your Essential Discoveries with some of the other students in your class and ask if they are helpful to them. You may want to revise your notes based on good ideas shared by your peers. Under Accomplishments, list at least three things you have accomplished since your last entry that relate to your career goals.

Discoveries:

_____
_____
_____
_____
_____
_____
_____
_____
_____
_____

Accomplishments:

_____
_____
_____
_____

BRAIDING & BRAID EXTENSIONS

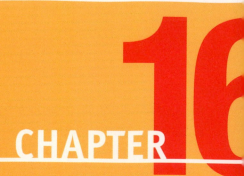

A Motivating Moment: "Everyone has his burden. What counts is how you carry it."—Merle Miller

After studying this chapter and completing the Essential Companion components, you should be able to:

1. Perform a client consultation and hair analysis with respect to hair braiding.

2. Explain how to prepare the hair for braiding.

3. Demonstrate the procedures for the invisible braid, rope braid, and fishtail braid.

4. Demonstrate the procedures for single braids, with and without extensions.

5. Demonstrate the procedures for cornrowing, with and without extensions.

ESSENTIAL BRAIDING

Why do I need to learn about braiding when I am not interested in providing these services?

Long hair styles with braids are becoming more and more popular across cultures, generations, and ethnic backgrounds. The fact is that many licensed cosmetologists do not offer these types of services. This can present a problem for clients desiring them. On the other hand, however, it can present an opportunity for those professionals who are expert in these services and readily available to provide them. By offering total hair care services to all clients, you will build a solid client base more readily and will never need to refer a client to another stylist or salon. In the end, you will reap the benefits of increased income and satisfied clients.

ESSENTIAL CONCEPTS

What do I need to know about braiding in order to provide a quality service?

In order to be properly prepared to offer quality braiding services, the first step you have to perfect is the client consultation. As with any service, learning to communicate with the client and truly listen to his or her desires, interests, and requests will be key in the success of the service. You will need to learn the important steps in preparing textured hair for braiding and/or hair extension services. Finally, you will need to be able to demonstrate masterful techniques for a wide variety of braids, including invisible, rope, fishtail, and single braids. You will want to perfect your skills in single braids and cornrowing, both with and without extensions. Once you have mastered these skills, you will have taken the first step in establishing a sound braiding business.

Preparing Textured Hair for Braiding

Number the following steps in their proper procedural order.

_____ Wash your hands.

_____ Gently towel-dry the hair.

_____ Gather required implements, materials, and supplies.

_____ Part damp hair from ear to ear across the crown. Use butterfly clips to separate the front section from back section.

_____ Shampoo, rinse, apply conditioner, and rinse thoroughly.

_____ Part back of head into four to six sections. Separate the sections with clips.

_____ Perform a client consultation and hair/scalp analysis.

_____ Beginning on the left section in the back, start combing the ends of the hair first, working your way up to the base of scalp. Lightly spray the section as you go along with detangling solution, if needed.

_____ Open one of the combed sections. Using fingers, apply blow-drying cream to hair from scalp to ends.

_____ Repeat steps 4 and 5 with the other sections of the hair until the entire head is sectioned.

_____ After combing thoroughly, divide section into two equal parts and twist them together to the end and hold section in place.

_____ Blow-dry using a pick nozzle attachment and hold hair down and away from the client's head as you begin drying. Use comb-out motion with the pick, always pointing the nozzle away from client.

_____ Place client under a medium heat hood dryer for five to ten minutes to remove excess moisture.

_____ Drape the client for a shampoo. If necessary, comb and detangle the hair.

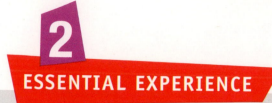

ESSENTIAL EXPERIENCE

The Developmental Stages of Locks

In the space provided, list all five phases in the development of locks in the left column. In the right column, thoroughly explain each phase.

STAGE	DEVELOPMENT

3

ESSENTIAL EXPERIENCE

Procedure for Basic Cornrows

Number the following steps in their proper procedural order (assume that the preparation segment has already been completed).

_____ **Repeat until all the hair is braided.** Apply oil sheen for a finished look.

_____ **Create a panel.** Start by taking two even partings to form a neat row for the cornrow base. With a tail comb, part the hair into a panel, using butterfly clips to keep the other hair pinned to either side.

_____ **Add new strands.** As new strands are added, the braid will become fuller. Braid to the end.

_____ **Cross the right strand.** Cross right strand (3) under the center strand (1). Passing the outer strands under the center strand this way creates the underhand cornrow braid.

_____ **Determine direction and size.** Depending on desired style, determine the correct size and direction of the cornrow base. With tail comb, part hair into 2-inch sections and apply a light essential oil to the scalp. Massage oil throughout scalp and hair,

_____ **Divide panel and cross left strand.** Divide the panel into three even strands. To ensure consistency, make sure strands are the same size. Place fingers close to the base. Cross the left strand (1) under the center strand (2). Center strand is now on the left and strand 1 is the new center.

_____ **Sanitation.** Follow clean-up and sanitation procedures for Invisible braid.

_____ **Continue braiding and add to outer strand.** As you move along the braid panel, pick up a strand from the scalp with each revolution and add it to the outer strand before crossing it under, alternating the side of the braid on which you pick up the hair.

_____ **Braid to ends.** Simply braiding to the ends can finish the cornrow; small rubber bands can be used to hold the ends in place. Other optional finishes, such as singeing, are considered advanced methods and require special training.

_____ **Add to outer strand.** With each crossing under, or revolution, pick up from the base of the panel a new strand of equal size and add it to the outer strand before crossing it under the center strand.

_____ **Braid next panel.** Braid the next panel in the same direction and in the same manner. Keep the partings clean and even.

4

ESSENTIAL EXPERIENCE

Word Search

After determining the correct words from the clues provided, locate the words in the word search puzzle.

Word	Clue
_____	Occurs after several years of maturation of a lock.
_____	Another name for cornrows.
_____	Narrow rows of visible braids that lie close to the scalp.
_____	Flat leather pads with close and fine teeth.
_____	Another name for locks.
_____	Simple two-strand braid in which hair is picked up from the sides and added to the strands as they are crossed over each other.
_____	The stage when a bulb can be felt at the end of each lock.
_____	A board of fine upright nails.
_____	Another name for visible braid.
_____	Three-strand braid produced by overlapping the strands of hair on top of each other.
_____	A manufactured synthetic fiber similar to coiled hair types.
_____	Beautiful wool fiber from Africa.
_____	Natural textured hair that is intertwined and meshed together to form a single or separate network.
_____	The phase of lock development when the lock is totally closed on the end.
_____	This method of locking takes advantage of the hair's natural ability to coil.
_____	In this stage of development, the hair is soft and coiled into spiral configurations.
_____	Braid made with two strands that are twisted around each other.
_____	Free-hanging braids, with or without extensions, that can be executed either underhand or overhand.
_____	This is the development of lock stage where hair begins to interlace and mesh.
_____	This refers to the hair diameter, feel, and wave pattern.
_____	Three-strand braid made by the underhand technique.
_____	Strong fiber from ox.

16

4

ESSENTIAL EXPERIENCE *continued*

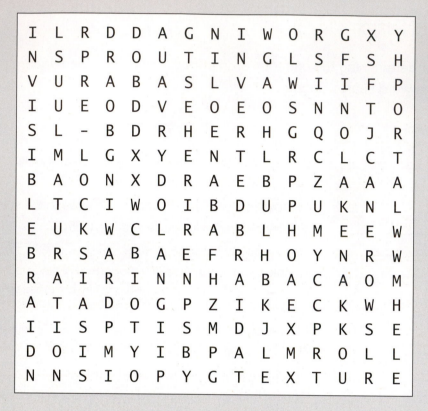

```
I L R D D A G N I W O R G X Y
N S P R O U T I N G L S F S H
V U R A B A S L V A W I I F P
I U E O D V E O E O S N N T O
S L - B D R H E R H G Q O J R
I M L G X Y E N T L R C L C T
B A O N X D R A E B P Z A A A
L T C I W O I B D U P U K N L
E U K W C L R A B L H M E E W
B R S A B A E F R H O Y N R W
R A I R I N N H A B A C A O M
A T A D O G P Z I K E C K W H
I I S P T I S M D J X P K S E
D O I M Y I B P A L M R O L L
N N S I O P Y G T E X T U R E
```

5

ESSENTIAL EXPERIENCE

Research and Design

Contact various salons in your area and interview them by asking the following questions.

- Does your salon offer braiding and/or extensions as a service?
- If yes, what braiding services do you offer?
- What braids are the most popular in your salon?
- What is the average time it takes your stylists to complete a full head of cornrows?
- What is the price structure your salon charges for braiding services?
- Do you have any specific advice for a newly licensed professional with respect to offering braiding services?

- Look through various style magazines and locate at least three different braided styles. Recreate those styles on a mannequin or a model.

- Use your imagination and the skills you have mastered in braiding to create a special effects braid. Stylists have created such looks as hats, flowers, baskets, or bird cages with braids. Tap into your creative abilities and design your own special look.

ESSENTIAL RUBRICS

Rubrics are used in education for organizing and interpreting data gathered from observations of student performance. It is a clearly developed scoring document used to differentiate between levels of development in a specific skill performance or behavior. A rubric is provided in this study guide as a self-assessment tool to aid you in your behavior development.

Rate your performance according to the following scale:

(1) Development Opportunity: There is little or no evidence of competency;
   Assistance is needed; Performance includes multiple errors.

(2) Fundamental: There is beginning evidence of competency;
   Task is completed alone; Performance includes few errors.

(3) Competent: There is detailed and consistent evidence of competency;
   Task is completed alone; Performance includes rare errors.

(4) Strength: There is detailed evidence of highly creative, inventive, mature presence of competency.

Space is provided for comments to assist you in improving your performance and achieving a higher rating.

INVISIBLE BRAID PROCEDURE

Performance Assessed	1	2	3	4	Improvement Plan
Pre-service sanitation and set up completed					
Performed client consultation					
Washed and sanitized hands					
Draped, shampooed, and dried hair					
Took triangular section at crown to hairline and divided into three equal strands, two in left, one in right					
Placed fingers close or away from scalp depending on desired tightness of braid					
Cross right strand over center strand, then crossed left over center strand					
Picked up 1" section of hair and added to center strand					
Switched hands and picked up 1" section on other side and continued braiding					
Moved down head with alternating pick-up movements					
Continued until braid was complete; secured with elastic band					
Accessorize as desired					
Post-service cleanup and appointment scheduling completed					

ESSENTIAL RUBRICS—CONT'D

ROPE BRAID PROCEDURE

Performance Assessed	1	2	3	4	Improvement Plan
Pre-service sanitation and set up completed					
Performed client consultation					
Washed and sanitized hands					
Draped, shampooed, and dried hair					
Took triangular section at crown to hairline and divided into three equal strands, two in left, one in right					
Divided hair into two equal strands; crossed right strand over left					
Placed both strands in right hand; twisted left strand two times clockwise					
Picked up 1" section from left side and added to left strand					
Placed both strands in left hand with palm up					
Picked up 1" section from right side and added to right strand					
Put both strands in right hand and twisted toward left					
Repeated sectioning and twisting procedure working toward nape until rope braid was finished					
Secured with an elastic band					
Post-service cleanup and appointment scheduling completed					

BASIC CORNROW PROCEDURE

Performance Assessed	1	2	3	4	Improvement Plan
Pre-service sanitation and set up completed					
Performed client consultation					
Washed and sanitized hands					
Draped, shampooed, and dried hair					
Parted hair into 2" sections and massaged in light oil					

ESSENTIAL RUBRICS—CONT'D

BASIC CORNROW PROCEDURE—cont'd

Performance Assessed	1	2	3	4	Improvement Plan
Took 2 even partings to form neat row for cornrow base					
Divided panel into 3 even strands					
Cross right strand under center strand					
With each revolution, picked up strand from scalp and added to outer strand before crossing it under					
Alternated side of head hair was picked up					
Braided to the ends to finish row; secured with elastic band					
Braided remainder of panels in same manner					
Repeated until all hair was braided					
Applied oil sheen for a finished look					
Post-service cleanup and appointment scheduling completed					

ESSENTIAL REVIEW

Using the following words, fill in the blanks below to form a thorough review of Chapter 16: Braiding. Words or terms may be used more than once or not at all.

box braids	double twisting	occupation	shorter
center strand	forehead	oval	small forehead
challenges	invisible	ox	softens
chemicals	jawline	palm roll	spiral
coil	length	partial bangs	configurations
coil pattern	locks	pomades	synthetic fiber
cornrows	matte finish	rope	temples
dampened	maturation	rope-like	visible
subsections	nails	rotating motion	
diameter	natural curl	round	
diffuser	network	several weeks	

1. Braiding styles have been known to distinguish one's tribe, age, economic status, _____ , geographic location, religious standing, and marital status.

2. Hair is referred to as "natural" or "virgin" if it has had no previous coloring or lightening treatments, _____ , or physical abuse.

3. Natural hairstyling uses no chemicals or tints and does not alter the _____ or coil pattern of the hair.

4. When referring to braiding and other natural hairstyling, the term *texture* refers to the _____ of the hair, the wave pattern of the hair, and the feel of the hair.

5. With regard to wave pattern, a _____ is a very tight curl pattern that is spiral in formation and, when lengthened or stretched, resembles a series of loops.

6. When styling with braids, add height to create the illusion of thinness for the _____ facial shape.

7. Most braided styles are appropriate for the _____ facial shape.

ESSENTIAL REVIEW *continued*

8. Create styles that are full around the forehead or _____ to help create a more oval appearance for the diamond facial shape.

9. To create the illusion of length and to soften facial lines for the square facial shape, choose styles that frame the face around the _____ , temples, and jawline.

10. Soft fringes around the forehead will camouflage a _____ without closing up the triangular-shaped face.

11. Creating full styles can make the oblong face shape appear _____ or wider.

12. The goals for the inverted triangle face shape is to minimize the width of the forehead by styling with _____ or wisps of hair/braids that frame the face.

13. A natural hairbrush, also known as a boar-bristle brush, is best for stimulating the scalp as well as removing dirt and lint from _____ .

14. The tool that dries the hair without disturbing the finished look and without removing moisture is called a _____ .

15. A board made of fine upright _____ through which human hair extensions are combed is called a hackle.

16. A manufactured _____ of excellent quality that has a texture similar to curly or coiled hair is called kanekalon.

17. A beautiful wool fiber imported from Africa has a _____ and comes only in black and brown is known as lin.

18. A strong fiber that comes from the domestic _____ found in the mountains of Tibet and Central Asia is yak.

19. _____ , gels, or lotions can be used to hold the hair in place for a finished look.

20. Textured hair, or hair with a tight _____ , presents certain challenges when styling because it is very fragile when both wet and dry.

21. Blow-drying the hair _____ it, makes it more manageable, loosens it, and elongates the wave pattern while stretching the hair shaft length.

22. Another term for a/an _____ braid is inverted.

23. The visible braid is a three-strand braid that employs the underhand technique, in which strands of hair are woven under the _____ .

24. A _____ braid is made with two strands that are twisted around each other.

25. Single braids, _____ , and individual braids are all considered to be free-hanging braids, with or without extensions, that can be extended with either an underhand or overhand stitch.

26. Narrow visible braids that lie close to the scalp are called _____ .

27. There are several ways to cultivate locks such as _____ , wrapping with cord, coiling, braiding, or simply by not combing or brushing.

28. Dreadlocks are natural textured hair that is intertwined and meshed together to form a single or separate _____ of hair and is done without the use of chemicals.

29. The method of placing the comb at the base of the scalp and, with a _____ , spiraling the hair into a curl is known as the comb technique.

30. The method that involves applying gel to _____ , placing the portion of hair between the palms of both hands, and rolling in a circular direction is known as palm roll.

31. Braids or extensions are an effective way to start locks and involve sectioning the hair for the desired lock and single braiding the hair to the end, with or without adding hair extensions and waiting for _____ of growth before employing the palm roll technique.

32. During the maturation stage of locks, the lock is totally closed at the end and the hair is tightly meshed, giving a _____ cylinder shape, except where there is new growth at the base.

33. During the pre-lock stage of locks, the hair is soft and coiled into _____ that are smooth and the end is open.

ESSENTIAL DISCOVERIES AND ACCOMPLISHMENTS

In the space below, jot some notes about what concepts of this chapter were hardest for you to understand or remember. Imagine finding yourself suddenly in the role of "teacher" and consider what you would tell your "students" about these difficult concepts. Share your Essential Discoveries with some of the other students in your class and ask if they are helpful to them. You may want to revise your notes based on good ideas shared by your peers. Under Accomplishments, list at least three things you have accomplished since your last entry that relate to your career goals.

Discoveries:

_____

_____

_____

_____

_____

_____

_____

_____

_____

_____

Accomplishments:

_____

_____

_____

_____

_____

WIGS & HAIR ENHANCEMENTS

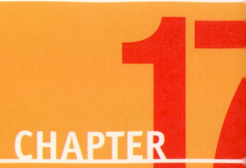

CHAPTER 17

A Motivating Moment: "A healthy attitude is contagious, but don't wait to catch it from others. Be a carrier!"—Unknown

ESSENTIAL OBJECTIVES

After studying this chapter and completing the Essential Companion components, you should be able to:

1. List the elements of a client consultation for wig services.

2. Explain the differences between human-hair and synthetic wigs.

3. Describe the two basic categories of wigs.

4. Demonstrate the procedure for taking wig measurements.

5. Demonstrate the procedure for putting on a wig.

6. Describe the various types of hairpieces and their uses.

7. Explain the various methods of attaching extensions.

ESSENTIAL ASPECTS OF WIGS AND HAIR ENHANCEMENTS

Do people really still wear wigs, and why should I know how to handle them?

Yes, people really do still wear wigs. They wear them for a number of reasons from convenience to need due to hair loss. Celebrities and people in the public eye, both male and female, wear wigs, hairpieces, or toupees, regularly to create a different, dramatic look. Like many other cosmetology services you will learn, the use of wigs has been prevalent throughout history from the early Egyptians to the present time. They became extremely popular again in the mid-20th century and continue to be used extensively in theater, music, and movie productions today.

You will also have clients from time to time who have medical problems or are undergoing chemotherapy treatments. As a result they may experience partial or total hair loss and will want to use wigs to maintain their personal appearance. You will need to be prepared to provide them the quality service they deserve, especially if they are experiencing a difficult time.

What can really be so hard about handling wigs, and what do I really need to know?

You need to know about the construction and materials used in wigs and how to care for each type of product, whether it is a human-hair piece or one constructed of synthetic hair. It will be important for you to know how to properly measure a client's head size and properly fit a wig. You will also want to master the special care needed for human-hair and hand-knotted wigs. Wigs that are made of human hair can also be colored to change the client's overall appearance. Hairpieces made of human hair can also be colored to blend with the client's own hair color as necessary. While this may not be the service that you spend the most time on, you will definitely want to be able to offer quality services to meet all your clients' needs.

1 ESSENTIAL EXPERIENCE

The History of Wigs

Conduct research about the history of wigs and write a brief essay on the subject. Be prepared to present the report to the full class if directed by your instructor. There are a number of resources you can refer to including the institution's library or resource center, encyclopedias, the Internet, and the community library. Obtain copies of pictures and prepare drawings to help illustrate your report.

_____

_____

_____

_____

_____

_____

_____

_____

_____

_____

_____

2
ESSENTIAL EXPERIENCE

Wig Measurements

Locate at least five models, and measure their heads for a wig. Use the following chart to record your findings.

Model Name					
Circumference					
Middle of forehead to nape					
Ear to ear across forehead					
Ear to ear over top of head					
Temple to temple across crown					
Width at nape line across nape of neck					

3 ESSENTIAL EXPERIENCE

Matching Exercise

Match each of the following essential terms with its definition.

_____ Turned hair

_____ Fusion

_____ Cascade regulation

_____ Capless wig

_____ Block

_____ Wiglet

_____ Full

_____ Hair extensions

_____ Switches

_____ Bonding

1. Strips of hair woven by hand or machine into long strips.

2. Hairpiece on an oblong base with curls or a cluster of curls that offers an endless variety of styling possibilities.

3. Section of hair, machine wefted on a round base, running across the back of the head.

4. Hair in which the roots and hair ends of all strands are aligned so that the cuticle slopes in the same direction.

5. Long wefts of hair mounted with a loop at the end.

6. Hair additions that are secured to the base of the client's natural hair in order to add length, volume, texture, or color.

7. Hairpiece with a flat, oblong base that fits on the top or back of the head.

8. Head-shaped form, usually made of canvas-covered cork or Styrofoam, to which the wig is secured for fitting, cleaning, coloring, and styling.

9. A machine-made wig in which rows of wefts are sewn to elastic strips in a circular pattern to fit the head shape.

10. Method of attaching extension in which the extension hair is bonded to the client's own hair with a bonding material that is activated by heat from a special tool.

4 ESSENTIAL EXPERIENCE

Crossword Puzzle

Clues:

Across

2. Method of attaching hair extensions with adhesive or glue gun
3. Wig consisting of elasticized mesh fiber to which hair is attached
6. Method of attaching extensions with bonding material activated by heat
7. Machine-made wig
9. Small wig used to cover top or crown of a man's head

Down

1. Hair addition that sits on top of hair and is usually attached by temporary methods
4. Hairpiece with an oblong base and curls or cluster of curls
5. Strip of hair woven by hand or machine onto a thread
8. Hairpiece consisting of a long length of wefted hair mounted with a loop on the end

5 ESSENTIAL EXPERIENCE

Windowpane—Wig Care

Windowpaning is the process of transferring key elements, points, or steps in a lesson into visual images that are hand sketched into the squares or "panes" of a matrix. Let your mind think in pictures and sketch the essential concepts printed in each of the following windowpanes. Don't be concerned with your artistic ability. Use lines and stick figures to depict the concepts requested.

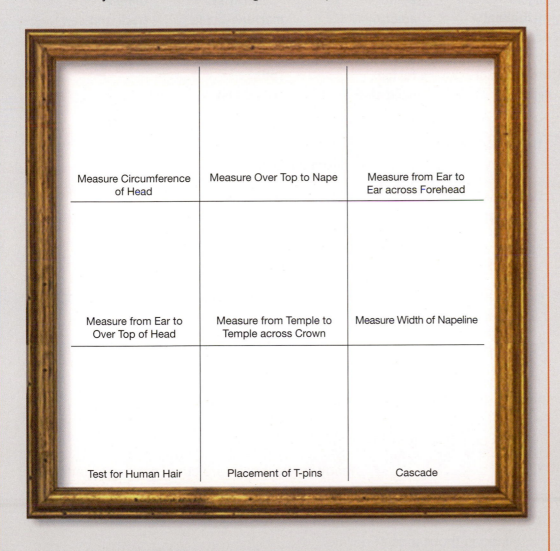

Measure Circumference of Head	Measure Over Top to Nape	Measure from Ear to Ear across Forehead
Measure from Ear to Over Top of Head	Measure from Temple to Temple across Crown	Measure Width of Napeline
Test for Human Hair	Placement of T-pins	Cascade

Using the following words, fill in the blanks below to form a thorough review of Chapter 17: Wigs and Hair Enhancements. Words or terms may be used more than once or not at all.

40%	cap wigs	human-hair	switch
60%	capless wigs	integration	synthetic
70%	cuticle-intact	key point	ten
angora	eight	checklist	toupee
attitudinal	emotional	machine-made	track-and-sew
boar bristles	film	oxidizing	weft
bonding	free-form	six	wig
bronze razors	fusion	split	
cap	hand-tied	strand test	

1. The ancient Egyptians shaved their heads with _____ and wore heavy wigs to protect them from the sun.

2. A wig service can be a large financial and _____ investment for a client.

3. Your best tool for achieving good communication during a wig consultation is to follow the _____

4. A _____ can be defined as an artificial covering for the head consisting of a network of interwoven hair.

5. One advantage of _____ wigs is they have the same styling and maintenance requirements as natural hair.

6. One disadvantage of human hair wigs is that the hair will break and _____ just like human hair if mistreated by harsh brushing, back combing, or excessive use of heat.

7. Most _____ ready-to-wear wigs are cut according to the latest styles, with the cut, color, and texture already set.

8. Well-crafted wigs, such as those used in _____ work, might be valued at thousands of dollars.

9. Animal hair that may be mixed with human hair to create a wig includes _____ , horse, yak, or sheep hair.

10. Hair that has been "turned" is also known as _____ hair.

ESSENTIAL REVIEW *continued*

11. _____ are constructed with an elasticized mesh-fiber base to which the hair is attached.

12. _____ are machine made with the hair woven into long strips called wefts.

13. _____ wigs are made by inserting individual strands of hair into a mesh foundation and knotting them with a needle.

14. _____ wigs are divided into three sections: the front edge, the side edge, and the back edge.

15. Canvas wig blocks are available in _____ sizes.

16. _____ cutting is usually done on dry hair, which allows you to see more clearly how the hair will fall.

17. Traditionally, brushes made with natural _____ have been regarded as the best on human hair.

18. Do not use _____ haircolor or haircolor with peroxide on wig hair that has been treated with metallic hair dye.

19. When coloring wigs or hairpieces, always _____ the hair prior to full color application.

20. A hairpiece gives 20% to _____ coverage and sits on top of the hair.

21. _____ hairpieces are very lightweight and natural looking, add length and volume to the client's hair, and allow the client's own hair to be pulled through and blended with the hair of the hairpiece.

22. A _____ is a small wig used to cover the top and crown of the head.

23. A _____ is a long length of wefted hair mounted with a loop on the end that covers 10%–20% of the head.

24. A wire-based hairpiece combines a hair _____ with a flexible wire.

25. In the _____ method, hair extensions are secured at the base of the client's own hair by sewing.

ESSENTIAL DISCOVERIES AND ACCOMPLISHMENTS

In the space below, jot some notes about what concepts of this chapter were hardest for you to understand or remember. Imagine finding yourself suddenly in the role of "teacher" and consider what you would tell your "students" about these difficult concepts. Share your Essential Discoveries with some of the other students in your class and ask if they are helpful to them. You may want to revise your notes based on good ideas shared by your peers. Under Accomplishments, list at least three things you have accomplished since your last entry that relate to your career goals.

Discoveries:

_____
_____
_____
_____
_____
_____
_____
_____

Accomplishments:

_____
_____
_____
_____
_____

CHEMICAL TEXTURE SERVICES

A Motivating Moment: "There are two big forces at work, external and internal. We have very little control over external forces such as tornados, earthquakes, floods, disasters, illness and pain. What really matters is the internal force. How do I respond to those disasters? Over that I have complete control." —Leo F. Buscaglia

ESSENTIAL OBJECTIVES

After studying this chapter and completing the Essential Companion components, you should be able to:

1. List the factors of a hair analysis for chemical texture services.

2. Explain the physical and chemical actions that take place during permanent waving.

3. List and describe the various types of permanent waving solutions.

4. Demonstrate base wrapping procedures: straight set, curvature wrap, bricklay wrap, weave wrap, double tool wrap, and spiral wrap.

5. Describe the procedure for chemical hair relaxing.

6. Understand the difference between hydroxide relaxers and thio relaxers.

7. Understand the difference between hydroxide neutralizers and thio neutralizers.

8. Explain the basic procedure for curl re-forming service.

ESSENTIAL CHEMICAL TEXTURE SERVICES

What role will permanent waving and hair relaxing have in my career when all I really want to do is style hair?

Actually, permanent waving, also known as a texture service, is the most popular chemical service offered in salons today. You will find that being able to provide your client with an appropriate texture service will improve your effectiveness as a hair designer. People have been trying to change the texture and curl of their hair since ancient Roman and Egyptian civilizations. Women wrapped their hair around sticks and men weaved their beards around them and then applied mud from the river which they allowed to dry in the sun for up to three days to achieve their desired look.

We've come a long way since those primitive methods. We began to make real progress in first part of the 20th century when Charles Nessler invented the permanent wave machine. Then in 1931 the pre-heat method of perming was introduced. The following year a method using external heat generated by chemical reaction was introduced. By 1941, the cold wave method was discovered, which used chemicals to soften and expand the hair and then re-harden it in its newly formed shape. This method does not use heat in any form. Technology continues to improve and new products are introduced regularly which allow the professional cosmetologist to modify the texture of a client's hair and render it more suitable for the desired style.

Our client culture has changed dramatically in the last few decades. Clients today want instant gratification from their salon visit and nearly all want better hair manageability. A texture service can play a huge role in helping the client manage his/her personal style between visits to the salon. Relaxers remove wave or curl from the hair in varying degrees. There is a large variety of hair types and individuals who will want the curl in their hair reduced. Hair relaxing services generate significant revenue for you and the salon. As a professional, you will want to be fully prepared to offer a quality service when it is requested.

Exactly what am I going to need to learn about permanent waving and chemical hair relaxing to be considered competent in this particular skill?

Your success in chemical texture services depends on your knowledge of the hair, your understanding of the chemicals used, and your ability to physically perform the service. Other factors relevant to the success of the service is the condition or integrity of the hair. The professional cosmetologist will know how to properly analyze a client's hair and scalp and select the appropriate products to create the desired look. You will also need to know how to select the correct tools and how to properly use them to "set" the perm. In addition, you need to prescribe the proper care of the chemical service to maintain its look for the maximum period of time.

Research and development of relaxer systems continues daily. As a result, we see state-of-the-art formulas and products available for our use in the salon. You will be exposed to these formulas while you are in school as well as in the professional establishment. Many manufacturers provide excellent education in the use of their products and you will want to take advantage of all that is available to you. In addition to product technology, you will want to learn all about the tools used in relaxing treatments as well as the procedures to follow to ensure success. As in perming, you must learn to conduct a thorough client consultation complete with hair and scalp analysis. Finally, you must master all the safety precautions that must be followed in this critical service.

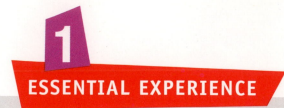

1

ESSENTIAL EXPERIENCE

Defining Permanent Waving and Identifying Textures

Permanent waving is a chemical and physical process in which the hair is wrapped around a rod, chemically softened and expanded, and finally chemically re-hardened into its newly formed shape.

In order to better understand the concept of texture, peruse old magazines (not beauty-industry related) for examples of different types of textures. You are not looking for texture that involves human hair. Cut out examples of the variety of textures and paste them in the space below, creating a texture collage. Beneath the collage, write a brief narrative describing the various textures selected and how they differ from each other.

_____

_____

_____

_____

2
ESSENTIAL EXPERIENCE

Hair Analysis

Choose three other students and perform a complete consultation and hair analysis on them. Fill out the school's client record card completely. Determine the correct rod size and product choice to create their desired textured look. Ask your instructor to review your record card and make an assessment as to the results you might achieve.

3
ESSENTIAL EXPERIENCE

Product Research

Research the various perm products used in your school. Make a chart of the products listing name, pH, key ingredients, and hair type for which they are recommended.

Product Name	Product pH	Key Ingredients	Hair Type

4

ESSENTIAL EXPERIENCE

Matching

Match the following essential terms with their identifying phrase or definition.

_____ Coarse texture

_____ Cortex

_____ Cuticle

_____ Fine texture

_____ Good porosity

_____ Medium texture

_____ Medulla

_____ Over porous

_____ Poor porosity

_____ Under processing

_____ Plastic cap

_____ Elasticity

_____ Density

_____ Body wave

_____ Waving lotion

_____ Book end

_____ Exothermic

_____ Croquignole

_____ End wraps

_____ Polypeptides

1. Result of over processing.

2. Processes more quickly than other textures.

3. Usually requires more processing than other textures.

4. Normal hair.

5. Resistant hair.

6. Innermost section of the hair.

7. Generally no problems processing.

8. Outer covering of the hair.

9. Major component of the hair structure.

10. Sulfite permanent.

11. One end paper folded over hair strand.

12. Hair ends wound from ends toward scalp.

13. The number of hairs per square inch.

14. The ability of the hair to stretch and contract.

15. Porous papers used to cover hair ends.

16. Heat is created chemically within the product.

17. Fits over the wrapped rods.

18. Amino acids are bonded together and form these.

19. Caused by insufficient processing time.

20. A liquid that softens and swells the hair.

5

Product Research

Research a variety of relaxer products available in your school and found at local supply stores. Use the chart below to track your findings.

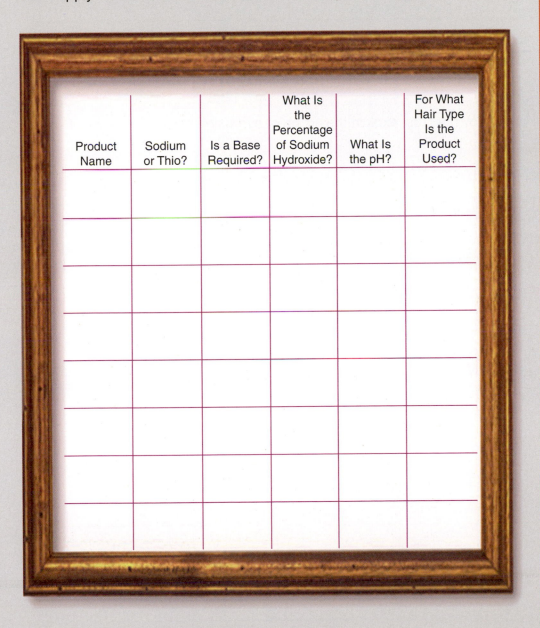

Product Name	Sodium or Thio?	Is a Base Required?	What Is the Percentage of Sodium Hydroxide?	What Is the pH?	For What Hair Type Is the Product Used?

6 ESSENTIAL EXPERIENCE

Purpose and Action of Chemical Hair Relaxing

List the products used in sodium hydroxide relaxers:

_____

_____

_____

In your own words, explain the action of hydroxide relaxers on the hair.

_____

_____

_____

_____

_____

What is the common ingredient in a thio type relaxer and permanent waving solution?

_____

Explain the action of this common ingredient.

_____

_____

_____

_____

6

ESSENTIAL EXPERIENCE *continued*

What is the purpose of the neutralizer in thio relaxing treatments?

_____

_____

_____

_____

In your own words, explain the difference between base and "no base" formulas, and the purpose of using a base product.

_____

_____

_____

_____

_____

_____

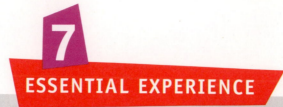

Word Search—Chemical Texture Services

After determining the correct words from the clues provided, locate the words in the word search puzzle.

Word	Clue
_____	Perm type having a pH between 7.8 and 8.2.
_____	Perm type having a pH between 9.0 and 9.6.
_____	Oily cream used to protect the skin and scalp during hair relaxing.
_____	Perm wrap in which one end paper is folded in half over hair ends.
_____	Rod having a smaller circumference in center than on ends.
_____	Hair strands are wrapped from ends to scalp.
_____	Partings and bases radiate throughout the panels to follow the curvature of the head.
_____	Side bonds between the polypeptide chains in the cortex.
_____	Waves activated by an outside heat source.
_____	Relatively weak physical side bonds resulting from an attraction between opposite electrical charges.
_____	Process by which hydroxide relaxers permanently straighten hair.
_____	Process of stopping the action of the permanent wave solution and hardening hair in new form.
_____	Also called end bonds.
_____	Relaxer having a pH above 10 and a higher concentration of ammonium thioglycolate.
_____	Wrapping technique that uses zigzag partings to divide base areas.

7 ESSENTIAL EXPERIENCE *continued*

```
G  N  C  E  Q  C  U  N  O  H  E  Y  E  D  S
H  E  O  N  W  U  B  O  J  F  R  I  I  M  D
Y  N  N  I  I  R  X  I  R  J  F  S  B  C  N
D  D  C  L  T  V  S  T  B  V  U  O  A  R  O
R  O  A  A  F  A  U  A  S  L  O  M  S  O  B
O  T  V  K  B  T  Z  Z  F  K  P  H  E  Q  E
G  H  E  L  K  U  P  I  E  B  O  W  C  U  D
E  E  R  A  M  R  D  N  L  V  C  A  R  I  I
N  R  O  S  X  E  D  O  T  A  O  O  E  G  T
B  M  D  G  B  W  Y  I  W  M  R  L  A  N  P
O  I  T  O  R  R  Z  H  U  E  J  T  M  O  E
N  C  N  A  F  A  D  T  Z  P  A  Q  U  L  P
D  D  P  O  E  P  G  N  B  D  K  V  B  E  I
S  A  C  I  D  -  B  A  L  A  N  C  E  D  N
F  N  N  R  E  X  A  L  E  R  O  I  H  T  X
```

ESSENTIAL RUBRICS

Rubrics are used in education for organizing and interpreting data gathered from observations of student performance. It is a clearly developed scoring document used to differentiate between levels of development in a specific skill performance or behavior. A rubric is provided in this study guide as a self-assessment tool to aid you in your behavior development.

Rate your performance according to the following scale:

(1) **Development Opportunity:** There is little or no evidence of competency; Assistance is needed; Performance includes multiple errors.

(2) **Fundamental:** There is beginning evidence of competency; Task is completed alone; Performance includes few errors.

(3) **Competent:** There is detailed and consistent evidence of competency; Task is completed alone; Performance includes rare errors.

(4) **Strength:** There is detailed evidence of highly creative, inventive, mature presence of competency.

Space is provided for comments to assist you in improving your performance and achieving a higher rating.

BASIC PERM WRAP PROCEDURE

Performance Assessed	1	2	3	4	Improvement Plan
Pre-service sanitation and set up completed					
Gathered products, materials, supplies, implements, and equipment					
Performed client consultation					
Washed and sanitized hands					
Draped, shampooed gently, and towel-dried hair					
Performed preliminary test curl					
Divided hair into 9 sections					
Began at hairline, made horizontal parting same size as rod, held hair at 90° angle.					
Used two end papers, rolled hair down to scalp, positioned tool half off base					
Bands were not twisted and were placed straight across top of tool					
Picks were inserted to stabilize rods and eliminate tension					
Continued wrapping remaining eight panels					
Applied barrier cream and cotton to hairline and ears					
Applied perm solution to each rod; followed directions plastic cap use					
Replaced saturated cotton					
Processed according to manufacturer's instructions and test curl					

ESSENTIAL RUBRICS—CONT'D

BASIC PERM WRAP PROCEDURE—cont'd

Performance Assessed	1	2	3	4	Improvement Plan
Rinsed thoroughly for 5 minutes; gently towel-blotted to remove excess moisture					
Applied neutralizer on each tool and timed according to directions					
Removed rods, worked neutralizer through hair and rinsed thoroughly					
Styled hair as desired					
Post-service cleanup and appointment scheduling completed					

CURVATURE PERM WRAP PROCEDURE

Performance Assessed	1	2	3	4	Improvement Plan
Pre-service sanitation and set up completed					
Gathered products, materials, supplies, implements, and equipment					
Performed client consultation					
Washed and sanitized hands					
Draped, shampooed gently, and towel-dried hair					
Combed hair in growth direction and sectioned to match length of rod					
Began wrapping first panel at hairline on one side of part with base away from face; used two end papers, rolled down half off base					
Remaining bases were slightly wider at end away from face; continued wrapping panel, alternating rod diameters					
Last rod in panel was directed up and toward base.					
Continue with panel two, three and so forth until wrap was complete					
Base direction contoured to perimeter hairline area					
Processed and neutralized according to directions					
Styled hair as desired					
Post-service cleanup and appointment scheduling completed					

BRICKLAY PERM WRAP PROCEDURE

Performance Assessed	1	2	3	4	Improvement Plan
Pre-service sanitation and set up completed					
Gathered products, materials, supplies, implements, and equipment					
Performed client consultation					
Washed and sanitized hands					
Draped, shampooed gently, and towel blotted hair					
Combed hair straight back and took section at front hairline the length and width of selected rod					
Held hair at 90° angle to head, using 2 end papers, rolled hair down to scalp and positioned rod half off-base					
Offset rod placement in subsequent rows in a bricklay pattern					
Continued to part out rows that radiated around curve of head through crown area					
Parted out horizontal sections in back of head continuing the bricklay pattern					
Processed and neutralized according to directions					
Styled hair as desired					
Post-service cleanup and appointment scheduling completed					

SPIRAL PERM WRAP PROCEDURE

Performance Assessed	1	2	3	4	Improvement Plan
Pre-service sanitation and set up completed					
Gathered products, materials, supplies, implements, and equipment					
Performed client consultation					
Washed and sanitized hands					
Draped, shampooed gently, and towel blotted hair					
Began at nape and worked toward top of head					

ESSENTIAL RUBRICS—CONT'D

SPIRAL PERM WRAP PROCEDURE—cont'd

Performance Assessed	1	2	3	4	Improvement Plan
Sectioned out first row along hairline at nape; combed remainder of hair up and secured out of way					
Parted out first base section; held hair at a 90° angle to head; using end papers began wrapping at one end of tool					
Rolled first two turns at a 90° angle to tool to secure ends; then spiraled hair on tool by changing angle; continued to spiral toward other end of tool; rolled hair down to scalp, positioned tool off base, secured by fastening ends of tool together					
Continued wrapping until first row was completed					
Sectioned out second row above and parallel to first row; combed remainder of hair up and secured it out of way					
Began wrapping at opposite side from where first row began and moved in the opposite directions established in first row					
Followed same procedure to wrap second row wrapping each tool at the opposite end established in first row					
Continued wrapping with same technique, in same direction, until second row was completed					
Sectioned out third row above and parallel to second row					
Followed same wrapping procedure, alternating rows from left to right while moving up the head					
Processed and neutralized hair according to directions					
Styled hair as desired					
Post-service cleanup and appointment scheduling completed					

VIRGIN HYDROXIDE OR THIO RELAXER PROCEDURE

Performance Assessed	1	2	3	4	Improvement Plan
Pre-service sanitation and set up completed					
Gathered products, materials, supplies, implements, and equipment					
Performed client consultation					

18

ESSENTIAL RUBRICS—CONT'D

VIRGIN HYDROXIDE OR THIO RELAXER PROCEDURE—cont'd

Performance Assessed	1	2	3	4	Improvement Plan
Washed and sanitized hands					
Draped client					
Parted hair into 4 sections					
Applied protective base					
Applied product first to top of strand then to underside in most resistant area making $\frac{1}{4}$" to 2" horizontal partings; applied $\frac{1}{4}$" to 2" away from scalp and up to porous ends					
Did not allow relaxer to touch scalp until last few minutes					
Continued application down toward hairline					
Continued same application procedure with remaining sections					
After applying relaxer, used back of comb or hands to smooth each section					
Processed according to manufacturer's directions; performed periodic strand tests					
During last few minutes of processing, worked relaxer down to scalp and through the ends of hair, using additional relaxer as needed; carefully combed and smoothed all sections					
Rinsed thoroughly with warm water to remove all traces of relaxer					
Neutralized according to directions, rinsed thoroughly, conditioned hair					
Styled hair as desired					
Post-service cleanup and appointment scheduling completed					

HYDROXIDE OR THIO RELAXER RETOUCH PROCEDURE

Performance Assessed	1	2	3	4	Improvement Plan
Pre-service sanitation and set up completed					
Gathered products, materials, supplies, implements, and equipment					
Performed client consultation					

18

ESSENTIAL RUBRICS—CONT'D

HYDROXIDE OR THIO RELAXER RETOUCH PROCEDURE—cont'd

Performance Assessed	1	2	3	4	Improvement Plan
Washed and sanitized hands					
Divide hair into four sections					
Applied protective base cream to hairline and ears					
Began application in most resistant area; made ¼" to 2" horizontal partings and applied relaxer to top of strand					
Applied relaxer ¼" to 2" away from scalp and only to new growth; did not allow relaxer to touch scalp until last few minutes of processing; did not overlap relaxer onto previously relaxed hair					
Continued applying relaxer using same procedure and working down section toward hairline					
Continued same application procedure in remaining sections					
After relaxer was applied to all sections, used back of comb or hands to smooth each section					
During last few minutes of processing, worked relaxer down to scalp					
If ends needed additional relaxing, worked relaxer through to ends for the last few minutes of processing only					
Rinsed thoroughly with warm water					
Followed virgin hydroxide neutralizing procedure					
Styled hair as desired					
Post-service cleanup and appointment scheduling completed					

SOFT CURL PERMANENT PROCEDURE

Performance Assessed	1	2	3	4	Improvement Plan
Pre-service sanitation and set up completed					
Gathered products, materials, supplies, implements, and equipment					
Completed client consultation					
Washed and sanitized hands					

ESSENTIAL RUBRICS—CONT'D

SOFT CURL PERMANENT PROCEDURE—cont'd

Performance Assessed	1	2	3	4	Improvement Plan
As an option, Draped, gently shampooed, towel-dried hair					
Parted hair into 4 sections					
Applied protective base cream to hairline and ears					
Began application in most resistant area; made $\frac{1}{4}$" to 2" horizontal partings and applied relaxer to top of strand first, then to underside					
Applied relaxer $\frac{1}{4}$" to 2" away from scalp up to porous ends; did not allow relaxer to touch scalp until the last few minutes of processing					
Continued application procedure through all sections					
After relaxer was applied to all sections, used back of comb or hands to smooth each section					
Processed according to directions; performed periodic strand tests					
During last few minutes of processing, worked the relaxer down to scalp and through to ends of hair; carefully combed and smoothed all sections					
Rinsed thoroughly with warm water to remove all traces of relaxer					
After rinsing hair, parted it into 9 panels; used length of rod to measure width of panels					
Wore gloves and wrapped most resistant area; applied distributed the thio curl booster to each panel; made a horizontal parting the same size rod					
Held hair at a 90° angle; used two end papers, rolled hair down and positioned rod half off-base.					
Continued wrapping remainder of panel and rest of hair using same technique					
Placed cotton around hairline and neck; applied thio curl booster to all curls until completely saturated; used cap properly					
Checked cotton and towels; processed according to directions; checked curl development by strand testing; rinsed thoroughly; towel blotted					

ESSENTIAL RUBRICS—CONT'D

SOFT CURL PERMANENT PROCEDURE—cont'd

Performance Assessed	1	2	3	4	Improvement Plan
Neutralized according to directions					
Styled hair as desired					
Post-service cleanup and appointment scheduling completed					

ESSENTIAL REVIEW

Complete the following review of Chapter 18: Chemical Texture Services by circling the correct answer to each question.

1. _____ rods have a small diameter in the center area and gradually increase to their largest diameter at the ends, resulting in a tighter curl at hair ends, with a loose, wider curl at the scalp.
   a) convex
   b) straight
   c) concave
   d) colored

2. A method of wrapping a permanent wave that is suitable for very long hair is the _____ .
   a) double halo method
   b) double tool technique
   c) single halo method
   d) straight back method

3. A _____ is an example of a physical change that results from breaking and re-forming the hydrogen bonds within the hair.
   a) blow-dry service
   b) wet set
   c) hair color service
   d) comb-out

4. All perm wraps begin by sectioning the hair into panels which are further divided into subsections called _____ .
   a) panels
   b) base sections
   c) base panels
   d) base control

5. Always rinse perm solution from the hair for at least _____ minutes before applying the neutralizer.
   a) 2
   b) 3
   c) 4
   d) 5

6. A/an _____ liquid protein conditioner can be applied to the hair and dried under a warm dryer for 5 minutes or more prior to neutralization if hair is damaged.
   a) alkaline
   b) emulsified
   c) neutral
   d) acidic

7. Ask _____ to find out why the client wants the texture service and what results are expected.
   a) open-ended questions
   b) close-ended questions
   c) rhetorical questions
   d) personal questions

ESSENTIAL REVIEW *continued*

8. Base control refers to the position of the tool in relation to its
_____ and is determined by the angle at which the hair is
wrapped.
   - a) panel
   - b) base section
   - c) base panel
   - d) scalp position

9. End wraps are absorbent papers used to _____ of the hair
when wrapping and winding hair on the perm tools.
   - a) decrease moisture
   - b) control ends
   - c) control elasticity
   - d) decrease elasticity

10. Hair texture describes the _____ of a single strand of hair and
is classified as fine, medium, or coarse.
   - a) length
   - b) color
   - c) curl
   - d) diameter

11. If the hair is not _____ , the hydrogen peroxide in the
neutralizer can react with waving lotion and cause the hair color to
lighten.
   - a) thoroughly shampooed
   - b) rinsed properly
   - c) lightly shampooed
   - d) lightly rinsed

12. If too many _____ bonds are broken in the perming process,
the hair will be too weak to hold a firm curl.
   - a) disulfide
   - b) hydrogen
   - c) salt
   - d) polypeptide

13. If you suspect metallic salts are present, mix 1 ounce of 20 volume
peroxide with 20 drops of 28% _____ and immerse at least 20
strands for 30 minutes.
   - a) bleach
   - b) hydrogen
   - c) ammonia
   - d) petroleum

14. If hair breaks under very slight strain, it has _____ .
   - a) excellent elasticity
   - b) very good elasticity
   - c) average elasticity
   - d) little or no elasticity

18

ESSENTIAL REVIEW *continued*

15. In order to make a smooth transition from the rolled section of the head to an unrolled section, use a larger tool for the last tool next to an unrolled section when giving a _____ .
    a) curvature perm
    b) partial perm
    c) spiral perm
    d) full perm

16. In neutralization, the bonds in the hair are re-formed _____ .
    a) immediately
    b) slowly
    c) sporadically
    d) randomly

17. In permanent waving, most of the processing takes place as soon as the solution penetrates the hair, within the first _____ minutes.
    a) 1 to 2
    b) 2 to 3
    c) 3 to 4
    d) 5 to 10

18. Many male clients are looking for added _____ , fullness, style, and low maintenance that only a perm can provide.
    a) color
    b) shine
    c) texture
    d) length

19. Metallic salts leave a coating on the hair that may cause _____ , severe discoloration, or hair breakage.
    a) mild odor
    b) uneven curls
    c) calcification
    d) smooth curls

20. Neutralization rebuilds the _____ by removing the extra hydrogen bonds created by the waving solution.
    a) salt bonds
    b) hydrogen bonds
    c) disulfide bonds
    d) polypetide chains

21. Perming only a section of a whole head of hair is called _____ .
    a) section perming
    b) spotmatic perming
    c) partial perming
    d) limited perming

22. Some manufacturers recommend the application of a _____ after blotting and before application of the neutralizer.
    a) pre-neutralizing conditioner
    b) pre-neutralizing shampoo
    c) post-processing moisturizer
    d) post-processing shampoo

ESSENTIAL REVIEW *continued*

23. The _____ wrap uses zigzag partings to divide base areas.
    a) curvature perm
    b) weave technique
    c) bricklay perm
    d) straight perm

24. The _____ wrap creates a movement that curves within sectioned-out panels.
    a) curvature perm
    b) bricklay perm
    c) weave technique
    d) straight perm

25. The basic perm wrap is also called a _____ wrap.
    a) curvature perm
    b) bricklay perm
    c) weave technique
    d) straight set

26. The chemical action of _____ breaks the disulfide bonds and softens the hair.
    a) ammonia
    b) hydrogen peroxide
    c) waving lotion
    d) neutralizer

27. The chemical composition of hair consists almost entirely of a protein material called _____ .
    a) polypeptides
    b) keratin
    c) cysteine
    d) melanin

28. Bonds that are formed between two cysteine amino acids located on neighboring polypeptide chains are _____ .
    a) salt
    b) chemical
    c) hydrogen
    d) disulfide

29. The polypeptide chains of this layer of hair are connected by end bonds and cross-linked by side bonds that form the fibers and structure of hair _____ .
    a) medulla
    b) cuticle
    c) cortex
    d) follicle

30. The perm that is activated by heat created chemically within the product is known as _____ .
    a) endothermic
    b) alkaline
    c) exothermic
    d) sodium hydroxide

18

ESSENTIAL REVIEW   *continued*

31. The action of waving lotion is to _____ .
    a) discolor the hair   b) shrink the hair
    c) expand the hair   d) condition the hair

32. The degree to which hair absorbs the waving lotion is related to its

    _____ .

    a) texture   b) length
    c) elasticity   d) porosity

33. The length of time required for the hair strands to absorb the waving lotion
    and for the hair to re-curl is called _____ .
    a) application time   b) processing time
    c) rinsing time   d) development time

34. The main active ingredient in acid-balanced waving lotions is

    _____ .

    a) glycerol monothioglycolate   b) ammonium thioglycolate
    c) hydrogen peroxide   d) sodium hydroxide

35. The main active ingredient or reducing agent in alkaline perms is

    _____ .

    a) glycerol monothioglycolate   b) ammonium thioglycolate
    c) hydrogen peroxide   d) sodium hydroxide

36. The _____ wrap is used to prevent noticeable splits and to blend
    the flow of the hair.
    a) curvature perm   b) bricklay perm
    c) spiral perm   d) basic perm

37. The _____ wrap is done at an angle that causes the hair to spiral
    along the length of the tool, like the grip on a tennis racquet.
    a) spiral   b) croquignole
    c) bricklay   d) barber pole

38. The hydrogen atoms in the disulfide bonds are so strongly attracted to the
    oxygen in the neutralizer that they release their bond with the sulfur atoms
    and join with the _____ .
    a) salt bond   b) nitrogen
    c) hydrogen   d) oxygen

ESSENTIAL REVIEW *continued*

39. Under processing is caused by _____ processing time of the waving lotion.
a) excessive
b) increasing
c) insufficient
d) exact

40. Waves that process more quickly and produce firmer curls than true acid waves are considered to be _____ .
a) alkaline
b) acid-balanced
c) ammonium thioglycolate
d) sodium hydroxide

41. What can be used to determine the actual processing time needed to achieve optimum curl results when giving a perm for the first time on a client?
a) patch test
b) strand test
c) porosity test
d) preliminary test curl

42. What type of hair is more fragile, easier to process, and more susceptible to damage from perm services?
a) coarse texture
b) medium texture
c) non-elastic
d) fine texture

43. What type of hair requires more processing than medium or fine hair and may also be more resistant to processing?
a) coarse texture
b) medium texture
c) non-elastic
d) fine texture

44. When the strand of hair is wrapped at an angle 45 degrees beyond perpendicular to its base section, it will result in _____ .
a) half-off base placement
b) off-base placement
c) on-base placement
d) on-stem placement

45. When one end paper is folded in half over the hair ends like an envelope, it is called the _____ .
a) double end paper wrap
b) book end wrap
c) single end paper wrap
d) top-hand wrap

46. When the strand of hair is wrapped at an angle 90 degrees (perpendicular) to its base section, it will result in _____ .
a) half-off base placement
b) off-base placement
c) on-base placement
d) on-stem placement

ESSENTIAL REVIEW *continued*

47. When performing a procedure for a preliminary test curl, wrap one tool in each different area of the head including the top, the side, and the _____.

a) bang
b) temple
c) nape
d) occipital

48. When hair has assumed the desired shape, the broken disulfide bonds must be _____ rebonded.

a) chemically
b) physically
c) temporarily
d) semi-permanently

49. When you place one end wrap on top of the hair strand and hold it flat, it is called the.

a) double flat wrap
b) bookend wrap
c) single flat wrap
d) top-hand wrap

50. A hair relaxing treatment should be avoided when an examination shows the presence of _____ .

a) scalp abrasions
b) strong curl
c) excessive oils
d) pityriasis steadoides

51. After saturating the rods with neutralizer in a soft curl permanent, the next step is to _____ .

a) rinse with hot water
b) remove rods carefully
c) completely dry hair
d) apply protective base

52. After the hair has been processed with a sodium hydroxide relaxer and before the shampoo, the hair should be thoroughly _____ .

a) oiled
b) rinsed
c) dried
d) conditioned

53. Before giving a relaxing treatment to overly curly hair, the cosmetologist must judge its texture, porosity, and _____ .

a) length and elasticity
b) elasticity and silkiness
c) elasticity and extent of damage, if any
d) softness and extent of damage, if any

continued

54. If using a "no base" relaxer, it is recommended that a protective cream be applied _____ .
a) at the nape of the neck
b) over the earlobes
c) the frontal hairline
d) on the hairline and around ears

55. Inspecting the action of the relaxer by stretching the strands to see how fast the natural curls are being removed is called _____ .
a) periodic patch testing
b) periodic relaxer testing
c) periodic strand testing
d) periodic elasticity testing

56. Of the general types of hair relaxers which one does not require pre-shampooing?
a) sodium hydroxide
b) sodium thioglycolate
c) ammonium thioglycolate
d) acid-based relaxers

57. One safety precaution for hair relaxing is to avoid _____ the scalp with the comb or fingernails.
a) massaging
b) scratching
c) smoothing
d) stimulating

58. Relaxers which are ionic compounds formed by a metal which is combined with oxygen and hydrogen are known as _____ .
a) guanidine hydroxide relaxers
b) metal hydroxide relaxers
c) low-pH relaxers
d) no-base relaxers

59. Sodium hydroxide relaxers are commonly called _____ .
a) guanidine hydroxide relaxers
b) low pH relaxers
c) lithium hydroxide relaxers
d) lye relaxers

60. The action of a sodium hydroxide relaxer causes the hair to _____ .
a) swell
b) shrink
c) harden
d) set

ESSENTIAL REVIEW *continued*

61. The process of breaking the hair's disulfide bonds during processing and converting them to lanthionine bonds when the relaxer is rinsed from the hair is known as _____ .
    a) lanolination
    b) lanthionization
    c) neutralization
    d) normalization

62. The scalp and skin are protected from possible burns when using a hair relaxer by applying _____ .
    a) cotton
    b) stabilizer
    c) base
    d) shampoo

63. The processing time of a chemical relaxer is affected by _____ .
    a) styling products used
    b) the client's age
    c) the hair's porosity
    d) brand of relaxer

64. The relaxer cream is applied near the scalp last because processing is accelerated in this area by _____ .
    a) body heat
    b) application speed
    c) body perspiration
    d) sebaceous glands

65. The chemical required to stop the action of the chemical relaxer is _____ .
    a) petroleum cream
    b) neutralizer
    c) conditioner
    d) waving lotion

66. The best type of shampoo to use after the chemical relaxer is _____ .
    a) an organic shampoo
    b) an antibacterial shampoo
    c) a neutralizing shampoo
    d) a dry shampoo

67. The strength of relaxer is determined by the strand test. General guidelines suggest that for coarse virgin hair, the following strength is used _____ .
    a) extra mild
    b) regular
    c) mild
    d) strong or super

ESSENTIAL REVIEW *continued*

68. The strength of relaxer is determined by the strand test. General guidelines suggest that for fine, tinted, or lightened hair, the following strength is used _____ .
a) extra mild
b) regular
c) mild
d) strong or super

69. The process of permanently rearranging the basic structure of overly curly hair into a straight form is called _____ .
a) thermal straightening
b) chemical hair relaxing
c) permanent waving
d) chemical hair softening

70. The combination of a thio relaxer and a thio permanent wrapped on large tools is called a _____ .
a) soft curl permanent
b) thioglycolate reconstructer
c) relaxer curl permanent
d) hard curl permanent

71. The most commonly used methods of hair relaxing are the sodium hydroxide method and the _____ method.
a) thermal
b) thio
c) ammonia
d) peroxide

72. To check relaxer processing, smooth and press a strand to the scalp using the back of the comb or your finger. If curl returns, _____ .
a) rinse immediately
b) add neutralizer
c) continue processing
d) add conditioner

73. What is used to restore the hair and scalp to their normal acidic pH?
a) cream conditioner
b) medicated shampoo
c) conditioning filler
d) normalizing lotion

74. What stops the action of any chemical relaxer that may remain in the hair after rinsing?
a) softener
b) breakdown cream
c) swelling compound
d) neutralizer

75. What are the two types of formulas for sodium hydroxide chemical hair relaxers?
a) base and no base
b) lye and no lye
c) stabilizer and no stabilizer
d) cream and no cream

18

76. What is one safety precaution that must be followed with all chemical hair relaxing services?
   a) shampooing the client's hair
   b) pre-conditioning the hair
   c) advising the client regarding processing time
   d) wearing protective gloves

77. What are the three basic steps used in chemical hair relaxing?
   a) wrapping, application, rinsing
   b) processing, neutralizing, conditioning
   c) shampooing, application, conditioning
   d) processing, neutralizing, stabilizing

78. When applying sodium hydroxide relaxer, the processing cream is applied last to the _____ and _____ .
   a) scalp area, middle of hair shaft
   b) scalp area, hair ends
   c) middle of hair shaft, hair ends
   d) nape area, hair ends

79. When performing a sodium hydroxide retouch, where is the product applied first.
   a) to the hair ends
   b) to the new growth only
   c) to middle of the hair shaft
   d) to the scalp area only

80. When using the comb method of application, how is the relaxing cream applied?
   a) with the back of the comb
   b) with the fingers
   c) with the applicator brush
   d) with the teeth of the comb

81. When processing is complete for a soft curl permanent, what is done after rinsing the hair thoroughly with warm water?
   a) each curl is blotted with towel
   b) conditioner is applied
   c) client is place under dryer
   d) test curl is taken

82. When hair has been sufficiently straightened, the hair is rinsed rapidly and thoroughly with _____ water.
   a) hot
   b) cold
   c) cool
   d) warm

ESSENTIAL DISCOVERIES AND ACCOMPLISHMENTS

In the space below, jot some notes about what concepts of this chapter were hardest for you to understand or remember. Imagine finding yourself suddenly in the role of "teacher" and consider what you would tell your "students" about these difficult concepts. Share your Essential Discoveries with some of the other students in your class and ask if they are helpful to them. You may want to revise your notes based on good ideas shared by your peers. Under Accomplishments, list at least three things you have accomplished since your last entry that relate to your career goals.

Discoveries:

_____

_____

_____

_____

_____

_____

_____

_____

_____

_____

Accomplishments:

_____

_____

_____

_____

_____

HAIRCOLORING

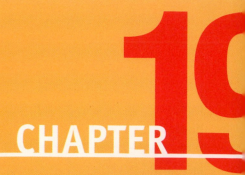

A Motivating Moment: "If you learn to appreciate more of what you already have, you will find yourself having more to appreciate."—Michael Angier

ESSENTIAL OBJECTIVES

After studying this chapter and completing the Essential Companion components, you should be able to:

1. Identify the principles of color theory and relate them to haircolor.

2. Explain level and tone and their role in formulating haircolor.

3. List the four basic categories of haircolor, explain their chemical effect on the hair, and give examples of their use.

4. Explain the action of lighteners.

5. Demonstrate the application techniques for (a) temporary colors, (b) semipermanent colors, (c) permanent colors, and (d) lighteners.

6. Demonstrate special effects haircoloring techniques.

ESSENTIAL HAIRCOLORING

Will I ever get over my fear of haircolor and be able to formulate and apply it successfully in the salon?

Without a doubt! Haircoloring is an art and you have just begun your training as an artist. This chapter is designed to help you begin to build your confidence with haircoloring in a practical and understandable way. Haircolor is considered to be the "cosmetic for the hair" in today's market. Your clientele are no longer afraid of haircolor and your haircolor clientele will range from teenage boys to grandmothers. By taking the time and effort required to learn haircolor, you will find that it is also a science as well as an art. You will learn that it is fun and easy and all your efforts will be rewarded financially in the salon.

What are the key concepts or elements in haircoloring that I need to know to be successful?

You will begin by learning about basic color theory, a refresher from what you learned in elementary school when you studied the colors of the rainbow. You will learn how to lighten dark hair to a light blond as well as how to darken lighter hair. You will learn about the reasons people color their hair and the psychological effects haircolor can have on an individual. You will learn about the Level System used by professionals and haircolor manufacturers to analyze the lightness or darkness of a color. As with any professional service, you will gain practice in performing a thorough client consultation prior to providing a haircolor service. You haircolor training will take you from temporary haircolor through semi-permanent, permanent, hair lightening, and special effects haircoloring procedures.

The Color Wheel

In the diagram below, place the colors that correspond with the color found on the wheel. You may use crayons, markers, colored pencils, water color paint, or cut the various colors out of magazines. Your goal is to depict the primary, secondary, and tertiary colors, and label each accordingly.

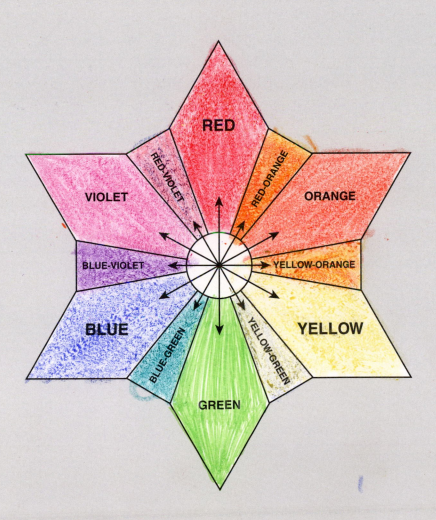

2

Haircolor Challenges/Corrective Solutions

In the grid below, explain the solutions to the haircoloring challenges listed.

Challenge	Solution
Yellowed Discoloration	— violet/purple
Resistant Gray Hair	— Permanet color (best for gray hair) / pre-softer.
Damaged Hair due to blow-drying, wind, harsh products, chemical services	— I wouldn't do anything semipermanent color. — Reconditioning treatmen
Damaged, Overly Porous Hair	— wouldn't do anything — use a conditioning fillers.
Red Hair	— Temporary hair color to — apropriate base color red orange / red violet / true red / Deposit only color
Brunette Hair	— temporary hair color — cool blue base — Do not lighten more than 2 levels.

Windowpane—Color Applications

Windowpaning is the process of transferring key elements, points, or steps in a lesson into visual images that are hand sketched into the squares or "panes" of a matrix. Let your mind think in pictures and sketch the essential concepts printed in each of the following windowpanes. Conduct additional research as applicable.

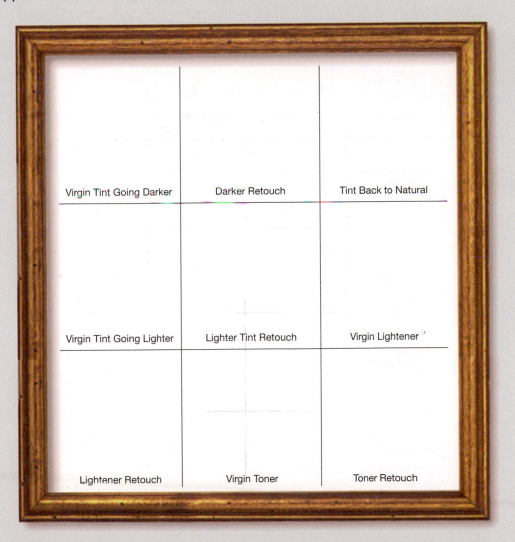

Virgin Tint Going Darker	Darker Retouch	Tint Back to Natural
Virgin Tint Going Lighter	Lighter Tint Retouch	Virgin Lightener
Lightener Retouch	Virgin Toner	Toner Retouch

6

ESSENTIAL EXPERIENCE

Crossword Puzzle—Haircolor

After identifying the appropriate word from the clues listed below, locate the word in the following crossword puzzle.

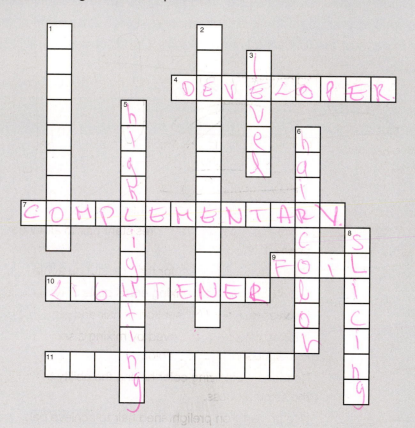

Clues:

Across

4. Oxidizing agent that mixes with an oxidation color and supplies oxygen gas
7. Colors opposite each other on the color wheel
9. Technique involving slicing or weaving out sections
10. Chemical compound for decolorizing hair
11. Color left in hair after it goes through ten stages of lightening

Down

1. Oxidizer added to hydrogen peroxide to increase chemical action
2. Used to treat gray or resistant hair
3. Unit of measurement of lightness or darkness of a color
5. Coloring some strands lighter than natural color
6. Industry term referring to artificial haircolor products
8. 1/8" section of hair positioned over foil

7 ESSENTIAL EXPERIENCE

Word Search—Haircolor

After identifying the appropriate words from the clues listed below, locate the words in the following word search puzzle.

Word	Clue
	Painting of lightener.
cap technique	Involves pulling hair through a perforated cap.
toner.	Used to ensure an even shade.
highlights	Coloring some strands lighter than natural color.
level.	Strength of color tone.
	Haircolor containing metal salts.
	First step in double-process haircoloring.
pre lightening	Process of treating gray or resistant hair to allow better penetration.
Primary	Pure or fundamental color than cannot be achieved by mixing.
Secondary	Color obtained from mixing equal parts of two primary colors.
Slicing	Involves taking a 1/8" section of hair and placing it on foil.
Tertiary	Intermediate color achieved by mixing a secondary color with its neighboring primary color.
	Permanent oxidizing color having the ability to lift and deposit in the same process.
Toner.	Use primarily on prelighted hair to achieve pale or delicate colors.
Volume-	The measure of varying strengths of hydrogen peroxide.
weaving.	Picking up strands with a zigzag motion of the comb.

19

7

ESSENTIAL EXPERIENCE *continued*

```
C R S F T V W S Y V F J K V H
A C E L G L C N A Y F X I I Y
P R E L I G H T E N I N G N N
T R M C L C Z L Q G F H T J N
E O E P E I I Q O P L Q K J M
C B T S T B F N R I Y H V A B
H M A L O W L I G H T I N G A
N W L G N F M H F Q I R F Y L
I T L P E A T H B R S O U V A
Q N I P R I S E C O N D A R Y
U K C Y N E M G N V E A R E G
E T O G G U Y R A I T R E T G
C H X E L W E A V I N G D Z E
G I V O I A P A U P I G O C E
L L V P N I G N O H T N C D T
```

8
ESSENTIAL EXPERIENCE

Matching Exercise—Haircolor

Match the following essential terms with their identifying phrase or definition.

_2._ Analysis   **1.** The predominant color and tone.

_3._ Blonding   **2.** An examination of the hair.

_6._ Coating   **3.** A term applied to lightening the hair.

_10._ Degree   **4.** Pigment that is fundamental and cannot be made.

_1._ Base color   **5.** The cuticle is lifted and the hair is overly porous.

_9._ Glaze   **6.** Residue left on the outside of the hair shaft.

_7._ Intensity   **7.** Strength of color tone

_5._ High porosity   **8.** Visible line separating colored hair from new growth.

_8._ Line of demarcation   **9.** A no lift deposit only color that adds shine and tone.

_4._ Primary color   **10.** Various units of measurement.

9

The Client Consultation

In the space provided below, list all the steps required in completing a thorough haircolor consultation. Then choose another student as your partner. Conduct a haircolor client consultation on each other. Record your results on the school's client record card and standard consultation form.

1. Do you want Enhance your hair color?

2. Blending or covering gray hair.

3. Lightening natural haircolor.

4. Depositing color on hair that has been lightened.

5. Creating Dimensional color

6. What is your natural hair color

7.

8.

9.

10.

ESSENTIAL RUBRICS

Rubrics are used in education for organizing and interpreting data gathered from observations of student performance. It is a clearly developed scoring document used to differentiate between levels of development in a specific skill performance or behavior. A rubric is provided in this study guide as a self-assessment tool to aid you in your behavior development.

Rate your performance according to the following scale:

(1) Development Opportunity: There is little or no evidence of competency; Assistance is needed; Performance includes multiple errors.

(2) Fundamental: There is beginning evidence of competency; Task is completed alone; Performance includes few errors.

(3) Competent: There is detailed and consistent evidence of competency; Task is completed alone; Performance includes rare errors.

(4) Strength: There is detailed evidence of highly creative, inventive, mature presence of competency.

Space is provided for comments to assist you in improving your performance and achieving a higher rating.

TEMPORARY HAIRCOLOR APPLICATION PROCEDURE

Performance Assessed	1	2	3	4	Improvement Plan
Pre-service sanitation and set up completed					
Gathered materials, implements, and supplies					
Performed client consultation					
Washed and sanitized hands					
Draped, shampooed and towel-dried hair					
Shook product, using gloves applied color and worked around head					
Used comb to blend; applied more color as needed					
Did not rinse; styled as desired					
Post-service cleanup and appointment scheduling completed					

SEMI-PERMANENT HAIRCOLOR APPLICATION PROCEDURE

Performance Assessed	1	2	3	4	Improvement Plan
Pre-service sanitation and set up completed					
Gathered materials, implements, and supplies					
Washed and sanitized hands					
Performed client consultation and scalp and hair analysis and recorded results					
Performed strand test					
Draped, shampooed and towel-dried hair; put on gloves					
Applied protective cream around hairline and ears					

SEMI-PERMANENT HAIRCOLOR APPLICATION PROCEDURE—cont'd

Performance Assessed	1	2	3	4	Improvement Plan
Applied color to entire hair shaft starting at scalp working gently through to ends					
Piled hair loosely and processed according to directions and strand test					
When developed, wet hair and worked into lather; rinsed thoroughly					
Shampooed gently, rinsed thoroughly and towel blotted hair					
Styled hair as desired					
Post-service cleanup and appointment scheduling completed					

SINGLE PROCESS COLOR FOR VIRGIN HAIR APPLICATION PROCEDURE

Performance Assessed	1	2	3	4	Improvement Plan
Pre-service sanitation and set up completed					
Performed preliminary strand test 24 to 48 hours prior to service; proceeded only if test was negative					
Washed and sanitized hands					
Performed client consultation and scalp and hair analysis; recorded results					
Draped client for haircolor service					
Applied protective cream around hairline and ears					
Parted dry hair into four sections					
Prepared tint formula for either bottle or brush application					
Began where color change would be greatest or where hair was most resistant. Parted off ¼" subsection with the applicator					
Lifted subsection and applied color to the mid-shaft area. Stayed at least 2" from the scalp, and did not go through the porous ends					
Processed according to strand test results. Checked color development by following the same steps used in strand testing					

19

ESSENTIAL RUBRICS—CONT'D

SINGLE PROCESS COLOR FOR VIRGIN HAIR APPLICATION PROCEDURE—cont'd

Performance Assessed	1	2	3	4	Improvement Plan
Applied color to the hair at the scalp.					
Pulled the color through onto the hair ends					
Lightly rinsed with lukewarm water; Massaged color into a lather and rinsed thoroughly					
Using a towel, gently removed any stains around hairline with shampoo or stain remover					
Shampooed hair; conditioned as needed					
Towel-dried and styled hair as desired					
Post-service cleanup and appointment scheduling completed					

SINGLE PROCESS TINT RETOUCH PROCEDURE

Performance Assessed	1	2	3	4	Improvement Plan
Pre-service sanitation and set up completed					
Performed preliminary strand test 24 to 48 hours prior to service; proceeded only if test was negative					
Washed and sanitized hands					
Performed client consultation and scalp and hair analysis; recorded results					
Draped client for haircolor service					
Applied protective cream around hairline and ears					
Parted dry hair into four sections					
Prepared tint formula for either bottle or brush application					
Applied tint to new growth only, being careful not to overlap on previously tinted hair					
Applied diluted color formula to the ends, according to analysis and strand test results					
Diluted remaining tint mixture with distilled water, shampoo, or conditioner					
Using a towel, gently removed any stains around hairline with shampoo or stain remover					

19

ESSENTIAL RUBRICS—CONT'D

SINGLE PROCESS TINT RETOUCH PROCEDURE—cont'd

Performance Assessed	1	2	3	4	Improvement Plan
Shampooed hair; conditioned as needed					
Towel-dried and styled hair as desired					
Post-service cleanup and appointment scheduling completed					

LIGHTENING VIRGIN HAIR PROCEDURE

Performance Assessed	1	2	3	4	Improvement Plan
Pre-service sanitation and set up completed					
Performed preliminary strand test 24 to 48 hours prior to service; proceeded only if test was negative					
Washed and sanitized hands					
Performed client consultation and scalp and hair analysis; recorded results					
Draped client for haircolor service					
Applied protective cream around hairline and ears					
Parted dry hair into four sections					
Prepared lightening formula and used immediately to prevent deterioration					
Wearing gloves, placed cotton strip at scalp area along parts to prevent lightener from touching base of hair					
Applied lightener at most resistant area; used $\frac{1}{8}$" partings and applied 2" from scalp and extended lightener only up to porous ends					
Applied lightener to top and underside of subsection in quick, rhythmic movements; completed all 4 sections					
Kept lightener moist; checked about 15 minutes prior to strand test results; reapplied product if necessary					
Continued checking until desired level was reached					
Removed cotton; applied lightener to hair near scalp with $\frac{1}{8}$" partings					
Processed and strand tested until entire shaft reached desired stage					
Rinsed thoroughly with tepid water; shampooed gently					

ESSENTIAL RUBRICS—CONT'D

LIGHTENING VIRGIN HAIR PROCEDURE—cont'd

Performance Assessed	1	2	3	4	Improvement Plan
Neutralized alkalinity with conditioner					
Towel-dried hair; examined scalp and analyzed condition of hair					
Proceeded with toner application if desired					

TONER APPLICATION PROCEDURE

Performance Assessed	1	2	3	4	Improvement Plan
Pre-service sanitation and set up completed					
Gathered and arranged materials, implements, and supplies					
Washed and sanitized hands					
Prelightened hair to desired stage of decolorization					
Shampooed hair lightly, rinsed, and towel-dried. Conditioned as necessary					
Selected desired toner shade					
Applied protective cream around hairline and over ears					
Took strand test and recorded results on client record card					
If using oxidative toner, mixed toner and developer in nonmetallic bowl or bottle, following manufacturer's directions					
Parted hair into four equal sections, using end of tail comb or tint brush. Avoided scratching scalp					
At crown of back quarter of head, parted of 1/4" partings and applied toner from scalp up to, but not including, porous ends					
Took strand test. If it indicated proper color development, gently worked toner through ends of hair, using brush or fingers					
If necessary for coverage, applied additional toner to hair and blended it in; Left hair loosely piled to permit air circulation or covered hair with cap if required					
Timed according to strand test. Checked frequently until desired shade was achieved					
Removed toner by wetting hair and massaging into a lather					

19

ESSENTIAL RUBRICS—CONT'D

TONER APPLICATION PROCEDURE—cont'd

Performance Assessed	1	2	3	4	Improvement Plan
Rinsed, shampooed gently, and rinsed well again					
Applied conditioner to close cuticle, lower the pH and help prevent fading					
Removed any toner stains from skin, hairline, and neck					
Styled as desired. Used caution to avoid stretching hair					
Post-service cleanup and appointment scheduling completed					

SPECIAL EFFECTS HAIRCOLORING WITH FOIL PROCEDURE

Performance Assessed	1	2	3	4	Improvement Plan
Pre-service sanitation and set up completed					
Gathered and arranged materials, implements, and supplies					
Washed and sanitized hands					
Performed preliminary strand test 24 to 48 hours prior to service; proceeded only if test was negative					
Performed client consultation and scalp and hair analysis; recorded results					
Draped client for haircolor service					
Applied protective cream around hairline and ears					
With a tail comb, took a slice of hair at the lower crown area of head					
Placed a piece of foil under the slice of hair					
Holding hair taut, brushed on lightener, from upper edge of foil to hair ends					
Holding hair taut, brushed on lightener, from upper edge of foil to hair ends					
Folded foil in half until ends meet					
Folded right side of foil in halfway, using comb to crease it. Then folded left side of foil in halfway					
Clipped foil upward					
Took a ¾" subsection in between foils. Clipped hair up and out of the way					

ESSENTIAL RUBRICS—CONT'D

SPECIAL EFFECTS HAIRCOLORING WITH FOIL PROCEDURE—cont'd

Performance Assessed	1	2	3	4	Improvement Plan
Continued working down back center of head until section was complete					
Once section was complete, released the clipped-up foils					
Working around head into side area, divided into two smaller sections					
Working down side, brought fine slices of hair into foil, applied lightener, clipped up foil					
Moved to other side of head and completed matching sections					
Moved to top of head. Took a fine slice of hair off top of a large section, placed on foil, and applied lightener					
Parted out larger section, took a fine slice from top of section, placed it on the foil, and applied lightener					
Continued toward front until last foil was placed					
Processed according to strand test. Checked foils to determine if desired level had been achieved					
Removed foils one at a time at shampoo area. Rinsed hair immediately to prevent color from affecting untreated hair					
Applied haircolor glaze to hair from base to ends					
Worked glaze into hair to ensure complete saturation. Processed up to 20 minutes					
Rinsed hair; shampooed and conditioned					
Styled hair as desired.					
Post-service cleanup and appointment scheduling completed					

ESSENTIAL REVIEW

Complete the following review of Chapter 19: Haircoloring by circling the correct answer to each question.

1. _____ are specialized preparations designed to help equalize porosity and deposit a base color in one application.
   - a) presofteners
   - b) color conditioners
   - c) conditioning activators
   - d) fillers ✓

2. A system for understanding the relationships of color is called _____.
   - a) the law of color
   - b) the level system
   - c) the color wheel ✓
   - d) primary color system

3. A _____ lightener is strong enough for high lift blonding, but gentle enough to use on the scalp.
   - a) oil
   - b) cream
   - c) powder ✓
   - d) paste

4. A product prepared by combining permanent haircolor, hydrogen peroxide, and shampoo is _____.
   - a) soap cap
   - b) highlighting shampoo ✓
   - c) color filler
   - d) highlighting shampoo tint

5. A mixture of shampoo and hydrogen peroxide creates a _____.
   - a) soap cap
   - b) highlighting shampoo
   - c) color filler ✓
   - d) highlighting shampoo tint

6. A no lift deposit only color that adds shine and tone to the hair is called a _____.
   - a) polish
   - b) wax
   - c) spray
   - d) glaze ✓

7. A process that lightens and colors hair in a single application is known as _____.
   - a) double-process haircoloring
   - b) temporary rinsing
   - c) single-process haircoloring ✓
   - d) virgin haircoloring

8. A patch test is generally conducted behind the ear or on the _____.
   - a) inner wrist
   - b) inner forearm
   - c) temple or forehead ✓
   - d) inside of the elbow

ESSENTIAL REVIEW *continued*

9. A combination of equal parts of prepared tint and shampoo that is applied to hair like regular shampoo is called a _____ .
   a) color filler
   b) hair presoftener
   c) soap cap
   d) shampoo tint

10. A/an _____ contains a powdered oxidizer that is added to hydrogen peroxide to increase its lifting power.
    a) activator
    b) protinator
    c) prohibitor
    d) developer

11. After the hair goes through the 10 stages of decolorizing, the color that is left in the hair is known as its _____ .
    a) foundation
    b) base
    c) vertex
    d) apex

12. An example of a natural or vegetable haircolor obtained from the leaves or bark of plants is _____ .
    a) henna
    b) tint
    c) toner
    d) demipermanent

13. Chemical compounds that lighten hair by dispersing, dissolving, and decolorizing the natural hair pigment are _____ .
    a) dispersers
    b) dissolvers
    c) decolorizers
    d) lighteners

14. Colored mousses and gels are considered to be what haircolor category?
    a) permanent
    b) semipermanent
    c) demipermanent
    d) temporary

15. Colors achieved by mixing equal parts of two primary colors are called _____ colors.
    a) secondary
    b) tertiary
    c) neutral
    d) protein

16. Colors tones that are golden, orange, red, and yellow are considered to be _____ tones.
    a) warm
    b) cool
    c) neutral
    d) primary

17. Colors tones that are blue, green, and violet are considered to be _____ tones.
    a) warm
    b) cool
    c) neutral
    d) primary

19

ESSENTIAL REVIEW *continued*

18. Equal parts of blue and yellow mixed together create _____ .
    a) pink
    b) violet
    c) green
    d) orange

19. Equal parts of red and yellow mixed together create _____ .
    a) pink
    b) violet
    c) green
    d) orange

20. Equal parts of red and blue mixed together create _____ .
    a) pink
    b) violet
    c) green
    d) orange

21. Hair texture is determined by the _____ of the individual hair strand.
    a) length
    b) strength
    c) diameter
    d) color

22. Haircolor that is able to deposit without lifting because they are less alkaline and are mixed with a low volume developer is _____ .
    a) permanent
    b) semipermanent
    c) demipermanent
    d) temporary

23. Haircolor that is mixed with a developer and remains in the hair shaft until the new growth of hair occurs is called _____ .
    a) permanent
    b) semipermanent
    c) demipermanent
    d) temporary

24. Haircoloring products fall into four classifications including temporary, semipermanent, and _____ .
    a) permanent and perpetual
    b) permanent and demipermanent
    c) demipermanent and perpetual
    d) vegetable and demipermanent

25. Metallic haircolors are also called _____ colors.
    a) advancing
    b) gradual
    c) delayed
    d) accelerated

26. One safety precaution in haircoloring is to never apply tint if _____ are present.
    a) parents
    b) children
    c) abrasions
    d) dandruff particles

27. Permanent haircolor is applied by either the bowl-and-brush method or with a/an _____ .
    a) spatula and brush
    b) applicator bottle
    c) bowl-and-bottle
    d) brush-and-bottle

28. Porous hair of the same color level will lighten faster than hair that is nonporous, because the bleaching agent can enter the _____ more rapidly.
    a) medulla
    b) cortex
    c) cuticle
    d) follicle

29. Primary and secondary colors that are positioned opposite each other on the color wheel are considered to be _____ .
    a) neutral
    b) complementary
    c) contradictory
    d) contrary

30. Products created to remove artificial pigment from the hair are known as _____ .
    a) color or tint removers
    b) pigment or melanin removers
    c) porosity removers
    d) highlight removers

31. The predominant tonality of an existing color is referred to as a _____ .
    a) base color
    b) even color
    c) neutral color
    d) deep color

32. The cortex or middle layer of the hair gives strength and elasticity and contributes about _____ % to the overall strength of the hair.
    a) 10
    b) 20
    c) 60
    d) 80

33. The strength of a color tone is referred to as _____ .
    a) level
    b) value
    c) depth
    d) intensity

34. The measure of the potential oxidation of varying strengths of hydrogen peroxide is _____ .
    a) density
    b) value
    c) volume
    d) percentage

19

ESSENTIAL REVIEW *continued*

35. The cuticle of the hair protects the interior and contributes _____ % to the overall strength of the hair.

a) 10
b) 20
c) 60
d) 80

36. The U.S. Federal Food, Drug, and Cosmetic Act prescribes that a patch test, also called a/an _____ test, be given 24 to 48 hours prior to an application of aniline derivative tint.

a) predisposition
b) allergy
c) reaction
d) postdisposition

37. The term used to describe the warmth or coolness of a color is _____ .

a) mixed melanin
b) contributing pigment
c) tone or tonality
d) value or depth

38. The preliminary strand test will tell you how the hair will react to the color formula and indicate _____ .

a) application method
b) processing time
c) client satisfaction
d) application time

39. The method used to analyze the lightness or darkness of a hair color, whether natural or artificial, is called _____ .

a) the law of color
b) the level system
c) the color wheel
d) primary color system

40. The tint formula in permanent haircolor contains uncolored dye _____ , which are small compounds that can diffuse into the hair shaft.

a) successors
b) precursors
c) activators
d) protinators

41. The melanin found in red hair is known as _____ .

a) pheomelanin
b) eumelanin
c) neomelanin
d) euromelanin

42. The melanin that gives black and brown color to hair is known as _____ .

a) pheomelanin
b) eumelanin
c) neomelanin
d) euromelanin

ESSENTIAL REVIEW *continued*

43. The ability of the hair to absorb moisture is called _____ .
    a) density
    b) texture
    c) elasticity
    d) porosity

44. The haircolor that partially penetrates the hair shaft and stains the cuticle layer, slowly fading with each shampoo, is known as _____ .
    a) permanent
    b) semipermanent
    c) demipermanent
    d) temporary

45. The number of hairs per square inch on the head relates to the hair's _____ .
    a) density
    b) texture
    c) elasticity
    d) porosity

46. The oxidizer that is added to hydrogen peroxide to increase its chemical action is known as the _____ .
    a) generator
    b) penetrator
    c) activator
    d) accelerator

47. The two methods of parting hair for a foil technique are _____ .
    a) slicing and striping
    b) weaving and striping
    c) slicing and threading
    d) slicing and weaving

48. The free-form technique of hair painting is also called _____ .
    a) toning
    b) baliage
    c) brushing
    d) swabbing

49. The first important guideline when color services do not turn out as planned or expected is _____ .
    a) call your instructor
    b) apply color rinse
    c) do not panic
    d) give money back

50. The system for understanding color relationships is the _____ .
    a) Level System
    b) Color System
    c) Law of Color
    d) Law of Hair

51. The process of treating gray or very resistant hair to allow for better penetration of color is known as _____ .
    a) presoftening
    b) prelightening
    c) activating
    d) accelerating

ESSENTIAL REVIEW *continued*

52. To some degree, the _____ is designed to protect the school or salon owner from responsibility for accidents or damages.
a) client record card
b) posted price list
c) release statement
d) indemnity insurance

53. What is added to hydrogen peroxide to increase its chemical action or lifting power?
a) accelerator
b) diffuser
c) dissolver
d) activator

54. What are the three types of hair lighteners?
a) oil, cream, powder
b) oil, paste, powder
c) cream, powder, paste
d) cream, paste, powder

55. What product is used to open the cuticle of the hair fiber so that tint can penetrate it?
a) hair conditioner
b) color filler
c) alkalizing agent
d) medicated shampoo

56. When performing retouches on red hair, the reds will last longer if you create them using a separate formula with a _____ haircolor product applied to the mid-shaft and ends of the strand.
a) high-lift
b) deposit-only
c) temporary
d) vegetable tint

57. When arranging for a haircolor service consultation, _____ walls are recommended.
a) pastel-colored
b) white or neutral
c) bright-colored
d) soft, yellow

58. When applying haircoloring products, always follow _____ .
a) manufacturer's directions
b) your instincts
c) client's directions
d) personal preference

59. Which type of lightener is not used directly on the scalp?
a) oil
b) cream
c) powder
d) paste

60. Which type of haircolor product uses the largest pigment molecules?
a) permanent
b) semipermanent
c) demipermanent
d) temporary

ESSENTIAL DISCOVERIES AND ACCOMPLISHMENTS

In the space below, jot some notes about what concepts of this chapter were hardest for you to understand or remember. Imagine finding yourself suddenly in the role of "teacher" and consider what you would tell your "students" about these difficult concepts. Share your Essential Discoveries with some of the other students in your class and ask if they are helpful to them. You may want to revise your notes based on good ideas shared by your peers. Under Accomplishments, list at least three things you have accomplished since your last entry that relate to your career goals.

Discoveries:

_____

_____

_____

_____

_____

_____

_____

_____

_____

Accomplishments:

_____

_____

_____

_____

SKIN DISEASES & DISORDERS

A Motivating Moment: "The big lesson of life is never be scared of anyone or anything. Fear is the enemy of logic."—Frank Sinatra

ESSENTIAL OBJECTIVES

After studying this chapter and completing the Essential Companion components, you should be able to:

1. Describe the aging process and the factors that influence aging of the skin.

2. Define important terms relating to skin disorders.

3. Discuss which skin disorders may be handled in the salon and which should be referred to a physician.

ESSENTIAL HISTOLOGY OF THE SKIN

Why do I need to learn about skin diseases and disorders when I really want to specialize as a hair designer?

As a practitioner in the field of cosmetology one of your primary responsibilities will be to help clients acquire and maintain healthy attractive skin, but not to actually diagnose skin disorders or diseases. However, becoming aware of basic clinical symptoms of various skin disorders will allow you to better serve your clients. If a condition is not serious, as a professional, you will be trained to make appropriate recommendations for controlling the condition. It is critical for you to be able to recognize those conditions that require a physician's care or might be infectious and spread disease from one person to another. So, yes, while you are not studying to become a dermatologist, having a thorough knowledge of the skin and its disorders will help you protect both your client and yourself from harm.

ESSENTIAL CONCEPTS

What do I need to know about the histology of the skin in order to perform professionally as a cosmetologist?

You need to become familiar with common disorders and diseases of the skin and recognize those conditions that cannot be treated or serviced by a cosmetologist. You will need to recognize the many disorders the skin can experience and know how to treat them. The chapter also contains a significant number of new terms and definitions that will be meaningful to you in your career as a cosmetologist.

Primary and Secondary Lesions

Write the definition of each of the primary and secondary lesions listed.

Macule _____

Papule _____

_____

Wheal _____

_____

Tubercle _____

_____

Tumor _____

_____

Vesicle _____

_____

Bulla _____

Pustule _____

Cyst _____

Scale _____

Crust _____

Excoriation _____

Fissure _____

Ulcer _____

Scar _____

_____

Keloid _____

Stain _____

_____

2

ESSENTIAL EXPERIENCE

Crossword Puzzle

Clues:

Across

2. Skin sore or abrasion from scratching or scraping
3. Blackhead
5. Excessive sweating
6. Deficiency in perspiration
7. Inflammatory skin condition
8. Protein that forms elastic tissue

Down

1. Foul-smelling perspiration
4. Dry, scaly skin caused by old age and exposure to cold

3

Crossword Puzzle

Clues:

Across

1. Inflammatory, painful itchy disease
4. Absence of melanin pigment
6. Study of skin
8. Crack in the skin
10. Chronic congestion on cheeks and nose
12. Large blister

Down

2. Protein giving skin form and strength
3. Outermost layer of skin
5. Increased skin pigmentation in spots
7. Malformation of skin due to abnormal pigmentation
9. Dead cells that form over a wound
11. Characterized by chronic inflammation of the sebaceous glands

4 ESSENTIAL EXPERIENCE

Word Search

Word	Clue
_____	Closed, abnormally developed sac, containing fluid, semifluid, or morbid matter, above or below the skin.
_____	Abnormal growth of the skin.
_____	Skin disorder characterized by light abnormal patches.
_____	Small, brownish spot or blemish on the skin.
_____	Inflamed pimple containing pus.
_____	Skin condition caused by abnormal increase of secretion from the sebaceous glands.
_____	Abnormal brown or wine-colored skin discoloration with a circular and irregular shape.
_____	Sebaceous cyst or fatty tumor.
_____	Abnormal rounded, solid lump above, within, or under the skin; larger than a papule.
_____	An abnormal cell mass resulting from excessive multiplication of cells, varying in size, shape, and color.
_____	Open lesion on the skin or mucous membrane of the body, accompanied by pus and loss of skin depth.
_____	Technical term for wart; hypertrophy of the papillae and epidermis.
_____	Milky-white spots (leukoderma) of the skin; acquired condition.
_____	Itchy, swollen lesion that lasts only a few hours; caused by a blow, an insect bite, urticaria, or the sting of nettle.

4 ESSENTIAL EXPERIENCE *continued*

```
K T S V F R E K G K B V Q A Y B C W
E N L K B C L D I A E L M L M I Y H
U P I U C K I X M R E O F V M D S E
Y L D A Q L H W R U T E Y A N T T A
M H C B T E Z U K A V C H X Y W V L
U Y Y E O S C O E I K Y Z O Q B I F
L R F P R A D T T B C E Q G O Z Y N
I U U M E E S I W C J J F I V I K U
R P E C R R L F V I Y I W Y S T F U
C O Z M R I T A G Y Z H R F E T J X
L Z A O G J A R E E W H C G V R W F
F U M O C G B G O H L E H X L O P L
B U N M V L N X Y P R C L P R R U K
T J K H O T G R Z E H R R U D W V Y
Z S E U D V I T A C F Y O E T U H K
E W O Q Q Y R U Q M B N M B B S T Z
H O Z P P R I Z W A Z Z R V E U U F
M O L E A G O B X T P H X D F S T P
```

ESSENTIAL REVIEW

Complete the following review of Chapter 20: Skin Diseases and Disorders by circling the correct answer to each question.

1. A condition of dry, scaly skin characterized by absolute or partial deficiency of sebum is _____ .
   a. rosacea
   b) asteatosis
   c) seborrhea
   d) steatoma

2. An itchy, swollen lesion that lasts only a few hours is a _____ .
   a) wheal
   b) tubercle
   c) bulla
   d) macule

3. When checking existing moles for signs of cancer, look for asymmetry, differences in size and shape, and changes in diameter and _____ .
   a) feel
   b) smell
   c) color
   d) symmetry

4. Smoking, drinking, taking drugs, and making poor dietary choices greatly influence the _____ process.
   a) developmental
   b) stimulation
   c) sunscreen
   d) aging

5. An abnormal rounded, solid lump above, within, or under the skin that is larger than a papule is known as a _____ .
   a) bulla
   b) cyst
   c) pustule
   d) tubercle

6. A thick scar resulting from excessive growth of fibrous tissue is a/an
   _____ .
   a) excoriation
   b) fissure
   c) ulcer
   d) keloid

7. Another name for a scar is _____ .
   a) crust
   b) excoriation
   c) ulcer
   d) cicatrix

8. A skin condition caused by an inflammation of the sebaceous glands is
   _____ .
   a) rosacea
   b) asteatosis
   c) seborrhea
   d) steatoma

ESSENTIAL REVIEW *continued*

9. A blister containing a watery fluid, similar to a vesicle, but larger, is a

   _____ .

   a) wheal   b) tubercle
   c) bulla   d) macula

10. A skin disease characterized by red patches, covered with silver white scales.

    a) eczema   b) psoriasis
    c) dermatitis   d) herpes simplex

11. An acquired, superficial, round, thickened patch of epidermis commonly know as callus, created by pressure or friction on the hands and feet, is a

    _____ .

    a) mole   b) freckle
    c) keratoma   d) verruca

12. Keratin-filled cysts that can appear just under the epidermis.

    a) milia   b) blackheads
    c) pimples   d) ulcers

13. An acute inflammatory disorder of the sweat glands, characterized by the eruption of small red vesicles and accompanied by burning, itching skin is known as _____ .

    a) steatoma   b) milia rubra
    c) hyperhidrosis   d) anhidrosis

14. A term used to indicate an inflammatory condition of the skin is

    _____ .

    a) eczema   b) psoriasis
    c) dermatitis   d) rosacea

15. An abnormal growth of the skin is called _____ .

    a) hypertrophy   b) hypertrichosis
    c) keratoma   d) callus

16. Foul-smelling perspiration is called _____ .

    a) anhidrosis   b) chloasma
    c) bromhidrosis   d) hypertrichosis

ESSENTIAL REVIEW *continued*

17. Deficiency in perspiration is called _____ .
    a) anhidrosis
    b) chloasma
    c) bromhidrosis
    d) hypertrichosis

18. A small brown or flesh-colored outgrowth of the skin is called a
    _____ .
    a) mole
    b) macule
    c) stain
    d) skin tag

19. An abnormal brown or wine-colored skin discoloration with a circular and irregular shape is called a _____ .
    a) mole
    b) macule
    c) stain
    d) skin tag

20. A spot or discoloration on the skin, such as a freckle, is called a
    _____ .
    a) mole
    b) macule
    c) stain
    d) skin tag

ESSENTIAL DISCOVERIES AND ACCOMPLISHMENTS

In the space below, jot some notes about what concepts of this chapter were hardest for you to understand or remember. Imagine finding yourself suddenly in the role of a teacher and consider what you would tell your students about these difficult concepts. Share your Essential Discoveries with some of the other students in your class and ask if they are helpful to them. You may want to revise your notes based on good ideas shared by your peers. Under Accomplishments, list at least three things you have accomplished since your last entry that relate to your career goals.

Discoveries:

_____

_____

_____

_____

_____

_____

_____

_____

_____

Accomplishments:

_____

_____

_____

_____

20

HAIR REMOVAL

CHAPTER 21

A Motivating Moment: "You can disagree without being disagreeable."—Zig Ziglar

ESSENTIAL OBJECTIVES

After studying this chapter and completing the Essential Companion components, you should be able to:

1. Describe the elements of a client consultation for hair removal.

2. Name the conditions that contraindicate hair removal in the salon.

3. List the two main classifications of hair removal and give examples of each.

4. Identify and describe three methods of permanent hair removal.

5. Demonstrate the techniques involved in temporary hair removal.

ESSENTIAL HAIR REMOVAL

Why do I need to learn about removing unwanted hair when I may never provide such a service?

The technical terms for superfluous hair are *hirsuties* (hur-SUE-shee-eez) and *hypertrichosis* (hy-pur-trī-KOH-sis). Actually, the terms mean nothing more than hair growth occurring in unusual amounts or locations on male and female clients. Often, those clients would like to have the hair removed and that's where the professional cosmetologist comes in. History documents that everything from abrasive pumice stones to sharpened stones and seashells have been used to rub off and pluck out hair. Records also indicate that the Egyptians made a compound of mud and alum for this purpose, and the Turks used a combination of yellow sulfide of arsenic, quicklime, and rose water, which created a primitive depilatory called rusma.

At some point nearly every client will encounter unwanted hair in one area or another. In fact, excessive hair can be extremely embarrassing and unattractive for female clients, especially when the hair is found on the face and chest. It is essential that you master the techniques used for removal of unwanted hair, and also learn to be sensitive when approaching a client about this type of service.

What do I need to know about hair removal in order to provide a quality service?

Hair removal falls into two major types: permanent and temporary, with salon techniques generally being limited to temporary methods. Permanent methods of hair removal include electrolysis, which is performed by a licensed electrologist, photo-epilation, and laser hair removal. Laws regarding photo-epilation and laser hair removal services vary in different states and provinces. However, the licensed cosmetologist should become proficient in all methods of temporary hair removal, including shaving (if allowed in your state or province), tweezing, using depilatories, and a variety of epilation techniques.

1 ESSENTIAL EXPERIENCE

Temporary and Permanent Methods of Hair Removal

In the space provided, identify the following methods of hair removal as either permanent or temporary.

Hot wax   _____

Shaving   _____

Electrolysis   _____

Tweezing   _____

Electronic tweezing   _____

Epilator   _____

Cold wax   _____

Photo-epilation   _____

Laser   _____

Depilatory   _____

Threading   _____

Sugaring   _____

2

Crossword Puzzle—Removing Unwanted Hair

Clues:

Across

1. Substance, usually a caustic alkali preparation, for temporary hair removal
3. Recommended when removing unwanted hair in large areas
5. Growth of an unusual amount of hair on parts of the body normally bearing only downy hair
9. Substance used to remove hair by pulling it out of the follicle
10. Temporary hair removal method that involves twisting and rolling cotton thread along the surface of the skin, entwining the hair in the thread and lifting it from the follicle
11. Temporary hair removal that involves the use of a thick, sugar-based paste

Down

2. A beam pulsed on the skin that impairs the hair follicle
4. Permanent hair removal treatment that uses intense light to destroy hair follicles
6. Advisable to determine whether the individual is sensitive to the action of the depilatory
7. Commonly used for shaping eyebrows
8. Hair removal by means of an electric current that destroys the hair root

2

ESSENTIAL EXPERIENCE *continued*

ESSENTIAL EXPERIENCE

Matching Exercise

Match the following essential terms with their identifying phrases or definition.

_____ Threading

_____ Cold wax

_____ Laser hair removal

_____ Tweezing

_____ Hot wax

_____ Electronic tweezing

_____ Epilator

_____ Shaving

_____ Sugaring

_____ Photo-epilation

1. Removes hair in large areas with razor and cream.

2. Depilatory that can be used on the cheeks, chin, upper lip, nape, arms, and legs.

3. Radio frequency transmits energy down the hair shaft into the follicle.

4. Used for clients who cannot tolerate heated wax.

5. A laser beam is pulsed on the skin, impairing the hair follicles.

6. Substance used to remove hair by pulling it out of the follicle.

7. The twisting and rolling of cotton thread along the skin surface, entwining the hair in the thread and lifting it from the follicle.

8. Commonly used for shaping the eyebrows.

9. Permanent hair removal treatment that uses intense light to destroy the hair follicles.

10. Temporary method of hair removal that uses a thick, sugar-based paste.

ESSENTIAL EXPERIENCE

Tweezing Eyebrows

Number the steps for an eyebrow tweezing procedure in the order in which the should occur.

Preparation: Tweezing Eyebrows

_____ Wash and dry hands and put on disposable gloves.

_____ Recline client as for facial. An alternative method is to seat client in a half-upright position and work from the side.

_____ Discuss type of arch suitable for facial characteristics.

_____ Drape towel over client's chest.

Procedure

_____ Use mild antiseptic on cotton ball prior to tweezing.

_____ Cleanse eyelid area. Use cotton balls moistened with gentle eye makeup remover.

_____ Remove hairs from above brow line. Brush hair downward. Shape upper section on one eyebrow; then the other. See Figure 21.13. Frequently sponge the area with antiseptic.

_____ Brush eyebrows to remove powder or scaliness. See Figure 21.10.

_____ Soften brows by saturating two cotton pledgets with warm water and place over brows for 1-2 minutes. See Figure 21.11. Surrounding skin may be softened with emollient cream.

_____ Remove hairs between brows by stretching skin taut with index finger and thumb on nondominant hand. Grasp each hair individually with tweezers and pull with a quick motion in the direction of hair growth. See Figure 21.12.
Tweeze between brows and above brow line first. The area under the brow line is much more sensitive.

_____ Remove hairs from under the brow line. Brush hairs upward. Shape the lower section of one brow, then the other. Sponge area with antiseptic.

_____ Sponge the tweezed area frequently with cotton moistened with an antiseptic lotion to avoid infection.

_____ Brush brow hair in its normal growth position.

_____ After tweezing, sponge brows and surrounding skin with astringent to contract the skin.

Cleanup and Sanitation

_____ Accompany client to reception area; suggest rebooking. Brows should be treated weekly.

_____ Continue makeup procedure if applicable.

_____ Remove towel and place in closed hamper.

_____ Wash hands with soap and warm water.

_____ Discard disposable materials in closed receptacle and disinfect implements.

ESSENTIAL RUBRICS

Rubrics are used in education for organizing and interpreting data gathered from observations of student performance. It is a clearly developed scoring document used to differentiate between levels of development in a specific skill performance or behavior. A rubric is provided in this study guide as a self-assessment tool to aid you in your behavior development.

Rate your performance according to the following scale:

(1) **Development Opportunity:** There is little or no evidence of competency; Assistance is needed; Performance includes multiple errors.

(2) **Fundamental:** There is beginning evidence of competency; Task is completed alone; Performance includes few errors.

(3) **Competent:** There is detailed and consistent evidence of competency; Task is completed alone; Performance includes rare errors.

(4) **Strength:** There is detailed evidence of highly creative, inventive, mature presence of competency.

Space is provided for comments to assist you in improving your performance and achieving a higher rating.

TWEEZING PROCEDURE

Performance Assessed	1	2	3	4	Improvement Plan
Pre-service sanitation and set up completed					
Performed client consultation					
Washed and sanitized hands					
Draped towel over client's chest; put on gloves					
Cleansed eyelid area with cotton balls moistened with eye makeup remover					
Brushed eyebrows to remove powder or scaliness					
Softened brows by saturating two cotton pledgets with warm water and place over brows for 1-2 minutes					
Used mild antiseptic on cotton ball prior to tweezing					
Removed hairs between brows by stretching skin taut; Grasped each hair individually with tweezers and pulled with a quick motion in direction of hair growth. Tweezed between brows and above brow line first.					
Sponged the tweezed area frequently with cotton moistened with an antiseptic lotion to avoid infection					
Removed hairs from above brow line. Brushed hair downward. Shaped upper section on one eyebrow; then the other. Frequently sponged the area with antiseptic.					
Removed hairs from under the brow line. Brushed hairs upward. Shaped the lower section of one brow, then the other. Sponged area with antiseptic.					

ESSENTIAL RUBRICS—CONT'D

TWEEZING PROCEDURE—cont'd

Performance Assessed	1	2	3	4	Improvement Plan
After tweezing, sponged brow area with astringent to contract the skin					
Brushed brow hair in its normal growth position					
Post-service cleanup and appointment scheduling completed					

HOT WAXING EYEBROWS PROCEDURE

Performance Assessed	1	2	3	4	Improvement Plan
Pre-service sanitation and set up completed					
Melted wax in heater (15-20 minutes)					
Completed client consultation.					
Laid clean towel over top of facial chair over a layer of disposable paper					
Placed hair cap or headband on client's head					
Draped towel over client's chest.					
Washed and dried hands and put on disposable gloves					
Removed makeup, cleansed area with mild astringent cleanser and dried					
Tested temperature and consistency of heated wax by applying small drop on wrist					
With spatula, spread thin coat of warm wax evenly over area to be treated, in direction OF hair growth. Did not put the spatula in the wax more than once.					
Applied sterile fabric strip over waxed area; pressed gently in direction of hair growth, running finger over surface of fabric three to five times					
Gently applied pressure to hold skin taut with one hand, quickly removed fabric strip and wax that sticks to it by pulling in direction opposite to hair growth. Did not pull straight up on strip.					
Lightly massaged treated area.					
Removed remaining wax residue from skin with gentle wax remover					

ESSENTIAL RUBRICS—CONT'D

HOT WAXING EYEBROWS PROCEDURE—cont'd

Performance Assessed	1	2	3	4	Improvement Plan
Repeated procedure on area around other eyebrow					
Cleansed skin with mild emollient cleanser and applied emollient or antiseptic lotion					
Removed headband and towel drape and place in closed hamper					
Post-service cleanup and appointment scheduling completed					

PROCEDURE

Performance Assessed	1	2	3	4	Improvement Plan
Pre-service sanitation and set up completed					
Melted wax in heater (15-20 minutes)					
Completed client consultation.					
Draped the treatment bed with disposable paper or a bed sheet with paper over the top					
If bikini waxing, offered the client disposable panties or a small sanitized towel					
If waxing the underarms, had the client remove her bra and put on a terry wrap. Offered a terry wrap when waxing the legs as well.					
Assisted the client onto the treatment bed and draped with towels.					
Washed hands with soap and warm water					
Thoroughly cleansed the area to be waxed with a mild astringent cleanser and dry					
Applied a light covering of powder.					
Tested the temperature and consistency of the heated wax by applying a small drop to wrist.					
Spread thin coat of the warm wax evenly over skin surface in same direction as hair growth. Did not put spatula in wax more than once. Removed stray wax with lotion to dissolve and remove wax.					
Applied sterile fabric strip in same direction as hair growth. Pressed gently, running hand over surface of fabric three to five times.					

21

PROCEDURE—cont'd

Performance Assessed	1	2	3	4	Improvement Plan
Gently applied pressure to hold the skin taut with one hand and quickly removed the adhering wax in the opposite direction of the hair growth.					
Applied gentle pressure and lightly massaged the treated area; repeated until service was complete.					
Had client turn over and repeated procedure on the backs of the legs.					
Removed remaining residue of powder from the skin.					
Cleansed area with a mild emollient cleanser and applied an emollient or antiseptic lotion.					
Undraped the client and escorted her to the dressing room.					
Post-service cleanup and appointment scheduling completed					

ESSENTIAL REVIEW

Using the words provided, fill in the blanks below to form a thorough review of Chapter 21: Hair Removal. Words or terms may be used more than once or not at all.

abrasions	electrolysis	opposite
acne	emollient	patch test
adhesives	epilator	radio frequency energy
allergies	eyebrows	rosacea
aloe gel	fever blisters	rusma
anagen	hydroquinone	sensitive
beeswax	hypertrichosis	shaving
botox	hypertrophy	steamed
client procedure	laser hair removal	strand test
collagen	needles	
depilatory	normal	

1. Another technical term for hirsuties is _____ .

2. A combination of yellow sulfide of arsenic, quicklime, and rose water that was used by the Turks as a crude hair removal agent is known as _____ .

3. A client consultation prior to a hair removal service discloses all medications, both topical and oral, along with any known skin disorders or _____ .

4. Facial waxing or tweezing should not be performed on clients who have _____ or very sensitive skin.

5. Having a history of _____ or cold sores is considered a contraindication for facial waxing.

6. Use of Retin-A, Renova, _____ , or similar products prevent hair removal treatments.

7. Removal of hair by means of an electric current that destroys the root of the hair is known as _____ .

8. Photo-epilation uses intense light to destroy hair follicles and has minimal side effects and requires no _____ .

21

ESSENTIAL REVIEW *continued*

9. A new method for the rapid, gentle removal of unwanted hair by means of a beam pulsed on the skin is called _____ .

10. Laser hair removal is most effective when used on follicles in the active growing phase, or _____ .

11. _____ is the most common form of temporary hair removal, particularly of men's facial hair.

12. Correctly shaped _____ have a strong, positive impact on the overall attractiveness of the face.

13. Washing your hands thoroughly with soap and warm water is critical before and after every _____ you perform.

14. When tweezing the eyebrows, tweeze between the brows and above the brow line first because the area under the brow line is much more _____ .

15. The method that transmits _____ down the hair shaft into the hair follicle are is called electronic tweezing.

16. Most manufacturers of electronic tweezers recommend that the area is _____ first in order to increase efficiency.

17. Depilatories contain detergents to strip the sebum from the hair and _____ to hold the chemicals to the hair shaft for the 5 to 10 minutes that are necessary to remove the hair.

18. If a client uses a chemical depilatory, you should perform a _____ to determine whether the individual is sensitive to the action of the product.

19. Wax is a commonly used _____ , applied in either hot or cold form as recommended by the manufacturer.

20. _____ has a relatively high incidence of allergic reaction.

21. When performing a wax service, the fabric strip and the wax that sticks to it are removed by pulling it in the direction _____ the hair growth.

22. Do not apply wax over warts, moles, _____ , or irritated or inflamed skin.

23. Apply _____ to calm and soothe sensitive skin that becomes red or swells due to a waxing procedure.

ESSENTIAL DISCOVERIES AND ACCOMPLISHMENTS

In the space below, jot some notes about what concepts of this chapter were hardest for you to understand or remember. Imagine finding yourself suddenly in the role of "teacher" and consider what you would tell your "students" about these difficult concepts. Share your Essential Discoveries with some of the other students in your class and ask if they are helpful to them. You may want to revise your notes based on good ideas shared by your peers. Under Accomplishments, list at least three things you have accomplished since your last entry that relate to your career goals.

Discoveries:

_____

_____

_____

_____

_____

_____

_____

_____

_____

_____

_____

Accomplishments:

_____

_____

_____

_____

_____

FACIALS

A Motivating Moment: "Yesterday is a dream, tomorrow but a vision. But today, well lived, makes every yesterday a dream of happiness, and every tomorrow a vision of hope. Look well, therefore to this day."—Sanskrit Proverb

ESSENTIAL OBJECTIVES

After studying this chapter and completing the Essential Companion components, you should be able to:

1. List and describe the different skin types and skin conditions.

2. Understand contraindications and the use of the health screening forms to safely perform facial treatments.

3. Identify the various types of massage movements and their physiological effects.

4. Describe different types of products used in facial treatments.

5. Understand the basic types of electrical equipment used in facial treatments.

6. Demonstrate the procedure for a basic facial.

ESSENTIAL THEORY OF MASSAGE

Why do I need to know about the underlying theory of massage, and are facials really that important in my career as a professional cosmetologist?

The term *massage* is of Arabic origin from the word *masa,* meaning to stroke or touch. The therapeutic benefits of massage were used and enjoyed in ancient Greece and are enjoyed more than ever today with the availability of licensed massage therapists. As a professional cosmetologist you will not only be given permission to invade the "comfort zones" of your clients, but you will be asked to actually touch them when you provide various services. For example, a good scalp massage can win the loyalty of your client for years to come. A massage that is both relaxing and stimulating accompanying a facial will inspire client confidence in you and will ensure repeat business. A firm massage given with flexible hands will ensure your clients receive the ultimate benefit from their services.

The generation born between the mid 1940s and the early 1960s is known as the baby boomer generation. As we enter the 21st century, that generation is growing older, ranging in age from their late 40s to their early 60s. With that aging of society, we have grown more interested in the health and beauty of the skin than ever before. Both men and women are buying more skin care products than ever before. The skin care industry is reported to be a multi-million dollar per year business. Professional advice and professional services are essential in ensuring optimum results for those men and women who want to keep their skin looking healthy and youthful. That's where you, the professional cosmetologist, come in. With your knowledge and practiced skills, you can provide the services they desire while also increasing your annual income significantly.

Remember that no matter how the benefits of a service are stressed, unless it is enjoyable to the client, the need and demand for the service will decline. A facial service that is accompanied by a good massage will endear you to your clients for years to come. A satisfied client means more clients and more satisfied clients means more income for you!

What to do I need to know about the theory of massage and facials in order to provide quality services to my clients?

It is essential that you master the basic manipulations used in massage in order to ensure a satisfactory service as well as to eliminate harm or injury to your client. It will be helpful for you to understand the psychological effects that a good massage will have on your clients. You will master numerous massage manipulations and become familiar with the motor nerve points of the face and the neck.

As a licensed cosmetologist, you will be able to perform many services relating to skin care and makeup. Among those services will be facials, facial massage, packs, and masks. It should be ever present in your mind that you are about to become a professional in the image industry. Therefore, it is essential that you exemplify that role. In addition to learning how to provide the best possible services for your clients, you must be a role model for the industry you represent. You must have the most current hairstyle, the most well-manicured hands and nails, and the best cared for skin. Once you have developed all the applicable skills in this specialty area, you will be in high demand for employment in the high-end, full-service salons in your marketplace.

1

Motor Nerve Points

On the diagrams below, identify the motor nerve points of the face and neck.

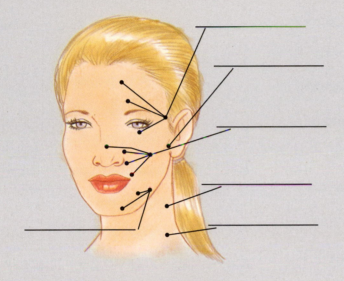

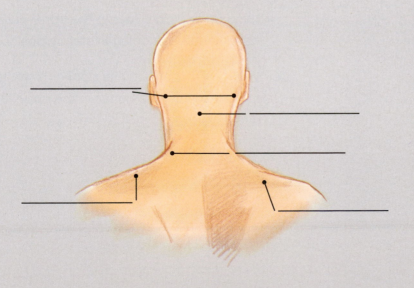

2 ESSENTIAL EXPERIENCE

Matching Exercise

Match the following essential terms with their identifying phrases or definition.

_____ Effleurage

_____ Petrissage

_____ Friction

_____ Percussion

_____ Vibration

_____ Rolling

_____ Chucking

_____ Wringing

_____ Tapotement

_____ Hacking

1. Tapping, slapping, and hacking movements.

2. Light, continuous, stroking movement.

3. Shaking movement.

4. Kneading movement.

5. Deep rubbing movement.

6. Chopping movement performed with edges of hands.

7. Another term for percussion.

8. Pressing and twisting the tissues with a fast back-and-forth movement.

9. Grasping flesh firmly in one hand and moving hand up and down along the bone while other hand keeps arm or leg in steady position.

10. Vigorous movement that applies a twisting motion against the bones in the opposite direction.

3
ESSENTIAL EXPERIENCE

Massage Manipulations

Label each of the manipulations found below in the space provided.

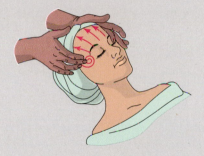

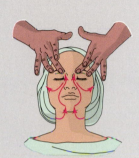

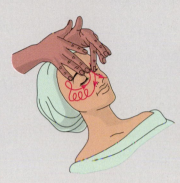

_____

_____

_____

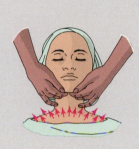

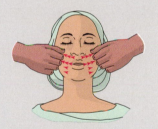

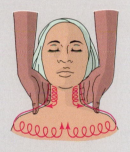

_____

_____

_____

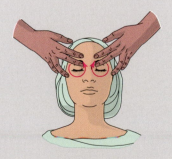

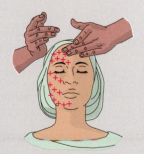

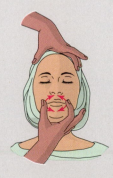

_____

_____

_____

4 ESSENTIAL EXPERIENCE

Word Scramble

Scramble	Correct Word
agreleueff	_ _ _ _ _ _ _ _ _ _ _
	Clue: Light, continuous stroking.
atenotempt	_ _ _ _ _ _ _ _ _ _
	Clue: Tapping, slapping, and hacking.
cepnoirssu	_ _ _ _ _ _ _ _ _ _
	Clue: Tapping, slapping, and hacking.
gilnflu	_ _ _ _ _ _ _
	Clue: Massaging the arms.
njtio	_ _ _ _ _
	Clue: Movable bone.
gmasesa	_ _ _ _ _ _ _
	Clue: Exercises facial muscles.
nbioitarv	_ _ _ _ _ _ _ _ _
	Clue: Shaking movement.
trmoo niopt	_ _ _ _ _ _ _ _ _ _
	Clue: Each muscle and nerve has one.
rcnfoiti	_ _ _ _ _ _ _ _
	Clue: Deep rubbing movement.
ragteissep	_ _ _ _ _ _ _ _ _ _
	Clue: Kneading movement.

5

ESSENTIAL EXPERIENCE

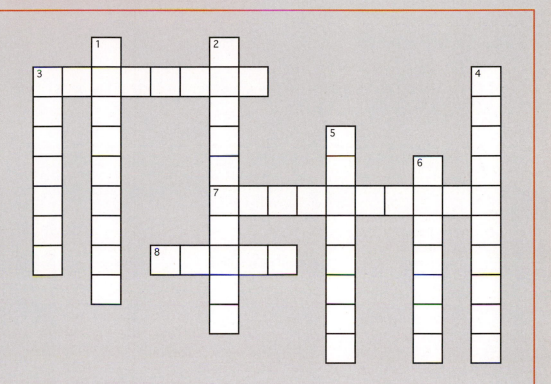

Clues:

Across
3. A deep rubbing movement
7. A kneading movement
8. Movable bone

Down
1. A shaking movement accomplished by rapid muscular contractions in your arm
2. Every muscle and nerve has one
3. A form of petrissage used mainly for massaging the arms
4. Light, continuous stroking movement applied with the fingers
5. A vigorous movement in which your hands are placed a short distance apart
6. Exercises facial muscles

6

Massage Movements

In the chart below, describe each massage movement, and list the parts of the body where the movement is used.

Name of Movement and Result Achieved	Movement Description	Where Used
Effleurage—		
Petrissage—		
Friction—		
Percussion—		
Vibration—		

7

ESSENTIAL EXPERIENCE

Word Scramble

Scramble	Correct Word
puekam atyr	_ _ _ _ _ _ _ _ _ _
nlaec thsee	_ _ _ _ _ _ _ _ _ _
laicaf eermtsa	_ _ _ _ _ _ _ _ _ _ _ _ _
askm	_ _ _ _
deah vocireng	_ _ _ _ _ _ _ _ _ _ _ _
eslwot	_ _ _ _ _ _
gsespno	_ _ _ _ _ _ _
ghhi qcyueerfn	_ _ _ _ _ _ _ _ _ _ _ _ _
itengtnrsa	_ _ _ _ _ _ _ _ _ _
fniredar mpal	_ _ _ _ _ _ _ _ _ _ _ _
ngifgniyam amlp	_ _ _ _ _ _ _ _ _ _ _ _ _ _ _
nolas wong	_ _ _ _ _ _ _ _ _
pslasuta	_ _ _ _ _ _ _ _
rireziutsom	_ _ _ _ _ _ _ _ _ _ _
scpiitenat	_ _ _ _ _ _ _ _ _ _
irbultacgni ilo	_ _ _ _ _ _ _ _ _ _ _ _ _ _
nottoc awssb	_ _ _ _ _ _ _ _ _ _ _
zuega	_ _ _ _ _

8 ESSENTIAL EXPERIENCE

Mind Map

Mind mapping creates a free-flowing outline of material or information. Using the central or key point of preservative and corrective facials, diagram the purpose and benefits of such treatments. Use terms, pictures, and symbols as desired. Using color will increase retention of the material. Keep your mind open and uncluttered and don't worry about where a line or word should go as the organization of the map will usually take care of itself.

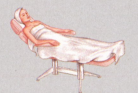

9

Client Consultation

Choose another student as your partner and conduct a facial treatment consultation on each other. Record your results on the sample record card found below. After the consultations, perform the appropriate facial service on each other. Ask an instructor to evaluate your procedure.

Department of Skin Care

Health Screening Form

Client History

Name_____

Address_____

City_____State_____Zip Code_____

Home phone_____ Work Phone_____

Occupation_____Referred by _____Date of Birth_____

Is this your first facial treatment?   YES____   NO____

Have you ever used:

Retin-A®?   YES____   NO____

Accutane®?   YES____   NO____

Are you using glycolic or alphahydroxy acids? YES____   NO____

Do you smoke? YES____   NO____

Are you pregnant? YES____   NO____

Do you have acne or frequent blemishes? YES____   NO____

Are you nursing? YES____   NO____

Taking birth control pills?   YES____   NO____   If so, how long?_____

Have you had skin cancer?   YES____   NO____

Do you experience stress? YES____   NO____   If so, how often?_____

Do you wear contact lenses?   YES____   NO____

Are you under a physician's care? YES____   NO____

Physician's Name_____

Do you have any allergies to cosmetics, foods, or drugs?   YES____   NO____

Please list_____

Are you presently on any medications - oral or topical-dermatological?   YES____   NO____

Please list_____

22

9 ESSENTIAL EXPERIENCE *continued*

What products do you use presently?_____

Please circle: Soap   Cleansing Milk   Toner   Daily Sunscreen   Creams

Other_____

Please circle if you are affected by or have any of the following:

Have had hysterectomy	Pacemaker/Cardiac Problems	Immune Disorders
Psychological	Herpes	Urinary or Kidney Problems
Taking Depression/Mood	Chronic Headaches	Hepatitis
Altering Medications	Fever Blisters	Lupus
Seborrhea/Psoriasis/Eczema	Metal Bone Pins or Plates	Epilepsy
Asthma	Sinus Problems	Other Skin Diseases
High Blood Pressure		

Please explain above problems or list any significant others:

_____

_____

I understand that the services offered are not a substitute for medical care, and any information provided by the therapist is for educational purposes only and not diagnostically prescriptive in nature. I understand that the information herein is to aid the therapist in giving better service and is completely confidential.

SALON POLICIES

1. Professional consultation is required before initial dispensing of products.

2. Our active discount rate is only effective for clients visiting every 4 weeks.

3. We do not give cash refunds.

I fully understand and agree to the above salon policies.

_____   _____

Client Signature   Date

10
ESSENTIAL EXPERIENCE

Crossword Puzzle

Clues:

Across
1. Correcting facial skin conditions
4. Used to help soften superficial
   lines and increase blood circulation
5. A disorder of the sebaceous
   glands
8. Maintains the health of the skin
9. Used to remove the product
   from containers
10. Whiteheads
11. Lamp used in facial treatments
13. May be made from vegetables,
   fruits, dairy products, herbs,
   and/or oils

Down
2. Blackheads
3. Used to hold the towel in place
6. Gauze used to hold certain
   mask ingredients on the face
7. Covering used to protect the
   hair
12. Skin type caused by insufficient
   flow of sebum

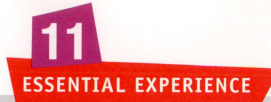

ESSENTIAL EXPERIENCE

Skin Care Product Research

Research a variety of skin care products available in your school and found at local supply stores. Include cleanser, toners, moisturizers, astringents, and so on. Use the chart below to track your findings.

Product Name	Pleasant Fragrance (Yes/No) Identify	Texture: How Does Product Feel?	Purpose of the Product	What Skin Type Is Product Used For

12

ESSENTIAL EXPERIENCE

Facial Steaming

Steaming the face can open pores, stimulate circulation, and help masks and creams work more effectively. Steaming should not be done more than once per week and should be accompanied by an appropriate moisturizer to avoid drying out the skin.

Try steaming at home by washing your face thoroughly and pinning or tying back your hair (or wear a shower cap). Boil a large pan of water and put in a handful of herbs based on your ingredient research. For example, chamomile, sage, peppermint, eucalyptus, and lavender disinfect and soothe the skin. They also contain oils that are beneficial to sinus passages. You can also use herbal oils from the health food store. Place the pan on a table or counter of appropriate height that will allow you to sit comfortably and hold your head over the pan. Lower your face over the pan and drape a large towel over your entire head and around the pan so no steam escapes. Now, relax and enjoy a highly rejuvenating experience. Steam for no more than 10 minutes. When finished blot your face with a soft cloth. Your skin is now prepared for an effective exfoliation or mask treatment. If not continuing with these treatments, refresh the skin with cool water to close the pores. In the space provided, record the results, your skin's reaction, and how the procedure made you feel.

_____

_____

_____

_____

_____

_____

_____

Rubrics are used in education for organizing and interpreting data gathered from observations of student performance. It is a clearly developed scoring document used to differentiate between levels of development in a specific skill performance or behavior. A rubric is provided in this study guide as a self-assessment tool to aid you in your behavior development.

Rate your performance according to the following scale:

(1) Development Opportunity: There is little or no evidence of competency; Assistance is needed; Performance includes multiple errors.

(2) Fundamental: There is beginning evidence of competency; Task is completed alone; Performance includes few errors.

(3) Competent: There is detailed and consistent evidence of competency; Task is completed alone; Performance includes rare errors.

(4) Strength: There is detailed evidence of highly creative, inventive, mature presence of competency.

Space is provided for comments to assist you in improving your performance and achieving a higher rating.

FACIAL MANIPULATIONS PROCEDURE

Performance Assessed	1	2	3	4	Improvement Plan
Performed facial pre-service preparation steps					
After sanitizing hands, applied massage cream					
Performed chin movement					
Performed lower cheek rotation movement					
Performed mouth, nose, and cheek movements					
Performed linear movement over forehead					
Performed circular movement over forehead					
Performed crisscross movement over forehead					
Performed stroking movement over forehead					
Performed brow and eye movement					
Performed nose and upper cheek movement					
Performed circular mouth and nose movement					
Performed lip and chin movement					
Performed lifting movement of cheeks					
Performed rotary movement of cheeks					
Performed light tapping movement					
Performed stroking movement of neck					
Performed circular movement over neck					

ESSENTIAL RUBRICS—CONT'D

FACIAL MANIPULATIONS PROCEDURE—cont'd

Performance Assessed	1	2	3	4	Improvement Plan
OPTIONAL MOVEMENTS Performed shoulders and back movement					
Performed back massage					
Repeated over shoulders and back to spine					
Remove cream; dusted back with talcum powder					
Proceed with additional desired services					
Post-service cleanup and appointment scheduling completed					

BASIC FACIAL WITH MASK PROCEDURE

Performance Assessed	1	2	3	4	Improvement Plan
Pre-service sanitation and set up completed					
Performed client consultation					
Washed and sanitized hands					
Properly draped chair and client					
Removed eye makeup					
Applied cleanser					
Removed cleanser residue					
Analyzed skin					
Steamed face					
Exfoliated face					
Applied massage cream, massaged face					
Removed massage cream					
Sponged face					
Applied treatment mask					
Removed mask					
Applied toner, astringent or freshener					

ESSENTIAL RUBRICS—CONT'D

BASIC FACIAL WITH MASK PROCEDURE—cont'd

Performance Assessed	1	2	3	4	Improvement Plan
Applied moisturizer					
Proceeded with additional desired services					
Post-service cleanup and appointment scheduling completed					

FACIAL FOR DRY SKIN PROCEDURE

Performance Assessed	1	2	3	4	Improvement Plan
Pre-service sanitation and set up completed					
Performed client consultation					
Washed and sanitized hands					
Properly draped chair and client					
Removed eye makeup					
Applied cleanser					
Removed cleanser residue					
Steamed face					
Exfoliated face					
Applied eye cream under eyes					
Applied moisturizer or massage cream					
Performed basic facial manipulations					
Removed massage cream					
Option #1 Performed galvanic treatment					
Option #2 Performed high frequency treatment					
Applied additional moisturizer					
Applied mask					
Applied cold cotton eye pads					
Removed mask					
Applied toner					

ESSENTIAL RUBRICS—CONT'D

FACIAL FOR DRY SKIN PROCEDURE—cont'd

Performance Assessed	1	2	3	4	Improvement Plan
Applied moisturizer or sunscreen					
Proceed with additional desired service					
Post-service cleanup and appointment scheduling completed					

FACIAL FOR OILY SKIN WITH OPEN COMEDONES PROCEDURE

Performance Assessed	1	2	3	4	Improvement Plan
Pre-service sanitation and set up completed					
Performed client consultation					
Washed and sanitized hands					
Properly draped chair and client					
Removed eye makeup					
Applied cleanser					
Removed cleanser residue					
Steamed face					
Exfoliated face					
Applied desincrustation lotion or gel					
Extracted comedones					
Applied astringent					
Applied high-frequency current					
If skin clogged, proceeded to mask step					
If not clogged, applied hydration fluid and performed massage manipulations					
Applied mask					
Removed mask					
Applied toner					
Applied moisturizer or sunscreen					

22

FACIAL FOR OILY SKIN WITH OPEN COMEDONES
PROCEDURE—cont'd

Performance Assessed	1	2	3	4	Improvement Plan
Proceeded with additional desired service					
Post-service cleanup and appointment scheduling completed					

FACIAL FOR ACNE-PRONE AND PROBLEM SKIN
PROCEDURE—cont'd

Performance Assessed	1	2	3	4	Improvement Plan
Pre-service sanitation and set up completed					
Performed client consultation					
Washed and sanitized hands					
Properly draped chair and client					
Removed eye makeup					
Applied cleanser					
Removed cleanser residue					
Steamed face					
Applied desincrustation lotion or gel and removed					
Extracted comedones					
Applied high-frequency treatment					
Applied positive galvanic current					
Performed facial massage manipulations					
Applied mask					
Removed mask					
Applied toner					
Applied moisturizer or sunscreen					
Proceeded with additional desired service					
Post-service cleanup and appointment scheduling completed					

ESSENTIAL REVIEW

Using the following words, fill in the blanks below to form a thorough review of Chapter 22: Facials. Words or terms may be used more than once or not at all.

5 to 7	enzyme peels	massage	preservative
7 to 10	essential oils	microdermabrasion	relaxation
astringents	exfoliation	modelage	rolling
clay masks	fresheners	moisturizers	soft hands
cleansing milk	from insertion to	motor	tonic lotions
cleansing lotion	origin	normal	treatment
client consultation	fulling	oily	vibration
combination	gauze	open skin pores	warm, moist
dehydration	gommage	origin	towels
dry	hacking movement	paraffin	wringing
effleurage	hands and arms	percussion	
emollients	massage cream	petrissage	

1. _____ creams are used to hydrate and condition the skin during the night when normal tissue repair is taking place.

2. _____ can be used to hold in place certain mask ingredients that tend to run.

3. _____ is a vigorous movement in which your hands are placed a little distance apart on both sides of the client's arm or leg. While working downward, a twisting motion is applied against the bones in the opposite direction.

4. _____ is used to achieve good slip during a massage.

5. A water-based emulsion that can be used twice daily on normal and combination skin for the purpose of removing makeup and soil is known as _____ .

6. A non-foaming lotion cleanser for the face is called _____ .

7. A light, continuous movement applied with fingers and palms in a slow, rhythmic manner without pressure is called _____ .

8. A form of petrissage in which the tissue is grasped, gently lifted, and spread out and used mainly on the arms is called _____ .

ESSENTIAL REVIEW *continued*

9. A shaking movement accomplished by rapid muscular contractions in the cosmetologist's arms, while the balls of the fingertips are pressed firmly on the point of application is known as _____ .

10. Oily or fatty ingredients that block moisture from leaving the skin are called _____ .

11. An enzyme peel in which a cream is applied to the skin before steaming and forms a hardened crust that is then massaged or "rolled" off the skin is called _____ .

12. Another name for chemical exfoliation procedures is _____ .

13. Aromatherapy refers to the therapeutic use of _____ .

14. Clay preparations used to stimulate circulation and temporarily contract the pores of the skin are _____ .

15. Cleansing cream is removed from the skin with tissues, moist cotton pads, facial sponges, or _____ .

16. Cosmetology services are generally limited to the scalp, face, neck, shoulders, upper chest, back, feet, lower legs, and _____ .

17. Every muscle and nerve has a _____ point which is the point over the muscle where pressure or stimulation will cause contraction of the muscle.

18. Fresheners, tonics, and astringents are all used to remove excess cleansers and residue left behind by face wash cleansers and are called _____ .

19. In addition to a firm sure touch and strong flexible hands, quality massage requires self-control and _____ .

20. Maintaining the health of the facial skin by using correct cleansing methods, increasing circulation, relaxing the nerves, and activating the skin glands and metabolism through massage is known as _____ facial treatments.

ESSENTIAL REVIEW *continued*

21. Masks that are melted at a little more than body temperature before application are _____ masks.

22. Masks that contain special crystals of gypsum that harden when mixed with cold water immediately before application are _____ masks.

23. Examples of mechanical exfoliants that work physically by "bumping off" dead cell buildup are granular scrubs, roll-off masks, and the use of _____ .

24. Skin that may have either oily and normal areas or normal and dry areas is known as _____ .

25. Skin that is lacking in oil and often dehydrated is considered to be _____ .

26. Skin that has an overabundance of sebum is considered to be _____ .

27. Skin that is usually in good condition and has an adequate supply of sebum and moisture is considered to be _____ .

28. Steam the face mildly with warm, moist towels or with a facial steamer in order to _____ .

29. The fixed attachment of one end of the muscle to a bone or tissue is called the _____ of muscles.

30. The most stimulating form of massage that is performed by tapping, slapping, or hacking movements is called _____ or tapotement.

31. _____ and astringents are usually stronger products, often with higher alcohol content, and are used to treat oilier skin types.

32. The manual or mechanical manipulation of the body by various movements to increase metabolism and circulation, promote absorption, and relieve pain is _____ .

ESSENTIAL REVIEW *continued*

33. The direction of massage movements should always be _____ .

34. The result achieved through light but firm, slow rhythmic movements, or very slow, light hand vibrations over the motor points for a short time is _____ .

35. The _____ movement involves pressing and twisting the tissues with a fast back-and-forth movement.

36. The condition that causes skin to feel dry and flaky because of an insufficient amount of water in the body is _____ .

37. The first step of all facial treatments is the _____ .

38. Use of the wrists and outer edges of hands in fast, light, firm, flexible motions against the skin in alternate succession is called _____ .

39. Water-based emulsions that are absorbed quickly without leaving any residue on the skin surface are called _____ .

40. When the skin is grasped between the fingers and palms and tissues are lifted from the underlying structures and squeezed, rolled, or pinched with light, firm pressure, it is called _____ .

ESSENTIAL DISCOVERIES AND ACCOMPLISHMENTS

In the space below, jot some notes about what concepts of this chapter were hardest for you to understand or remember. Imagine finding yourself suddenly in the role of "teacher" and consider what you would tell your "students" about these difficult concepts. Share your Essential Discoveries with some of the other students in your class and ask if they are helpful to them. You may want to revise your notes based on good ideas shared by your peers. Under Accomplishments, list at least three things you have accomplished since your last entry that relate to your career goals.

Discoveries:

_____

_____

_____

_____

_____

_____

_____

_____

_____

_____

_____

Accomplishments:

_____

_____

_____

_____

_____

FACIAL MAKEUP

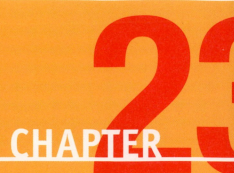

A Motivating Moment: "Keep your face to the sunshine and you cannot see the shadow."—Helen Adams Keller

ESSENTIAL OBJECTIVES

After studying this chapter and completing the Essential Companion components, you should be able to:

1. Describe the different types of cosmetics and their uses.

2. Demonstrate an understanding of cosmetic color theory.

3. Demonstrate a basic makeup procedure for any occasion.

4. Identify different facial types and demonstrate procedures for basic corrective makeup.

5. Demonstrate the application and removal of artificial lashes.

6. List safety measures to be followed during makeup application.

ESSENTIAL FACIAL MAKEUP

What makes applying makeup such a critical part of my career as a cosmetologist?

We've already discussed the fact that today's society is aging. As people age, they will do almost anything to feel and look younger. Women have the opportunity to apply makeup, which can do a great deal to emphasize their most attractive facial features and minimize those features that are not so attractive or are out of balance. Even though today's society places so much emphasis on this particular aspect of life, it is not a new concept. History shows that both men and women as far back as the New Stone Age used tattooing and body paint for ornamentation. Makeup has been used for tribal identification, religious ceremonies, preparation for war (remember Mel Gibson in the movie *Braveheart*), and a number of other occasions or events. The Egyptians were quite innovative and used a combination of ground alabaster or starch mixed with vegetable dyes and mineral salts.

We have Elizabeth Arden and Max Factor to thank for turning cosmetic makeup into an industry all its own back in the 1930s. Without a doubt cosmetic makeup is here to stay. For a cosmetologist, that means more opportunity and more money!

What to do I need to know about facial makeup in order to provide a quality service?

You need to consider the structure of the client's face, the color of the eyes, skin, and hair. You will need to consider how the client wants to look, keeping in mind the reasonable results you will be able to achieve. For example, you can't change a huge nose into a petite nose. You can, however, artistically and scientifically apply makeup and arrange hair so as to minimize the size of the nose. You will truly become an artist when you can apply color, shading, and highlighting to create illusions that present the client in the most attractive manner. You will need to know all the techniques used for face shapes and features, and, as a professional cosmetologist, you will be able to apply all those techniques combined with the appropriate hair color and design to create the best possible image for your client.

1 ESSENTIAL EXPERIENCE

Commercial Cosmetics

Choose a partner and conduct a joint research project. Your goal is to create a collage of commercial cosmetics in at least two categories, such as daytime makeup, evening makeup, normal skin, dry skin, or oily skin.

Look through industry and fashion magazines and choose ads that depict various types of cosmetics, such as lipstick, eye cream, moisturizer, foundation, mascara, etc. Cut out the ads, use colored markers, and any other implements to create an artistic representation for your chosen category.

Your collage, built on a large poster board or other suitable background, should depict a complete cosmetic and skin care regimen for the category you have chosen.

Be prepared to do an oral presentation to your classmates about your project, explaining each product's purpose and how it is used.

2 ESSENTIAL EXPERIENCE

Windowpane—Face Shapes

Windowpaning is the process of transferring key elements, points, or steps in a lesson into visual images that are hand sketched into the squares or "panes" of a matrix. Let your mind think in pictures and sketch the essential concepts printed in each of the following windowpanes. Don't be concerned with your artistic ability. Use lines and stick figures to depict the concepts requested.

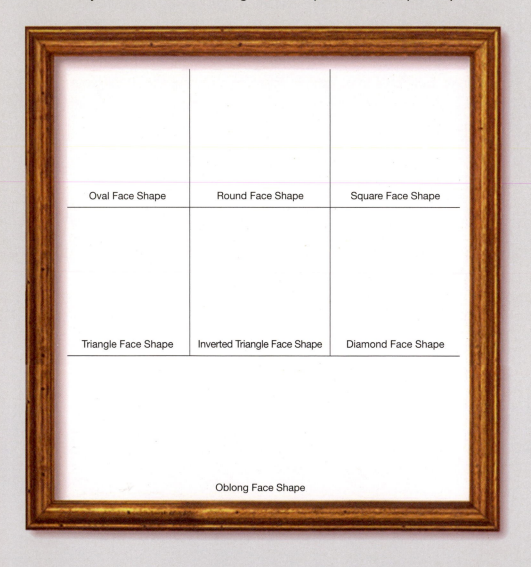

Oval Face Shape	Round Face Shape	Square Face Shape
Triangle Face Shape	Inverted Triangle Face Shape	Diamond Face Shape
	Oblong Face Shape	

3
ESSENTIAL EXPERIENCE

Word Scramble

Scramble	Correct Word
ragel sone	＿＿＿＿＿＿ ＿＿＿＿
	Clue: Apply a darker foundation on the nose and a lighter foundation on the cheeks at the sides of the nose
talf seon	＿＿＿＿＿ ＿＿＿＿
	Clue: Apply a lighter foundation down the center of the nose, stopping at the tip
esolc tes seye	＿＿＿＿＿＿ ＿＿＿ ＿＿＿＿
	Clue: Apply shadow lightly up from the outer edge of the eyes
wanorr jnaliwe	＿＿＿＿＿＿＿ ＿＿＿＿＿＿＿＿
	Clue: Highlight by using a lighter shade foundation over the prominent area of the jawline
ayveh dilded	＿＿＿＿＿＿ ＿＿＿＿＿＿＿
	Clue: Shadow evenly and lightly across the lid from the edge of the eyelash line to the small crease in the eye socket
tsorh chtik nekc	＿＿＿＿＿＿ ＿＿＿＿＿＿ ＿＿＿＿＿
	Clue: Use a darker foundation on the neck than the one used on the face
doarb osen	＿＿＿＿＿＿ ＿＿＿＿＿
	Clue: Use a darker foundation on the side of the nose and nostrils
wedi tes	＿＿＿＿ ＿＿＿
	Clue: Extend brow lines to inside corners of the eye
doabr wajenil	＿＿＿＿＿＿ ＿＿＿＿＿＿＿＿
	Clue: Apply a darker shade of foundation over the heavy area of the jaw, starting at the temples

3

ESSENTIAL EXPERIENCE *continued*

ugnibgl yees   ＿ ＿ ＿ ＿ ＿ ＿ ＿ ＿ ＿ ＿ ＿

Clue: Minimize by blending the shadow carefully over the prominent part of the upper lid

gnol niht kcne   ＿ ＿ ＿ ＿ ＿ ＿ ＿ ＿ ＿ ＿ ＿ ＿

Clue: Apply a lighter shade foundation on the neck than the one used on the face

dnuor seye   ＿ ＿ ＿ ＿ ＿ ＿ ＿ ＿ ＿ ＿

Clue: Lengthen by extending the shadow beyond the outer corner of the eyes

4

Corrective Lip Treatment

On the diagrams below, use colored pencils to illustrate how lipstick can be applied to create the illusion of more balanced and proportioned lips.

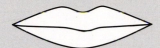

Thin lower lip

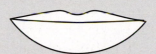

Thin upper lip

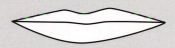

Thin lips

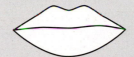

Small mouth

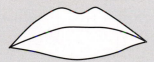

Drooping corners

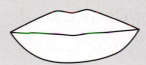

Oval lips

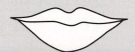

Sharp peaks

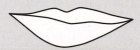

Uneven lips

Crossword Puzzle

Clues:

Across

2. Part of a complete and effective makeup application if well-groomed
5. Used to remove makeup from containers
6. Individual artificial eyelashes
8. Base or protective film
10. Used to remove excess facial hair
11. Used to add matte finish to face

Down

1. Used for theatrical purposes
3. Used to accentuate eyelids
4. Used to color cheeks
7. Used to cover blemishes
9. Used to darken, define, and thicken lashes

6

Band Lash Procedure

Number the following steps in the preparation, procedure, and cleanup activities for applying artificial band eyelashes in the order they should occur.

Preparation

_____ Wash your hands.

_____ Drape client. Properly drape the client to protect her clothing and have her use a hairline strip, headband, or turban during the procedure.

_____ Remove eye makeup. If the client has not already done so, remove all eye makeup so that the lash adhesive will adhere properly. Work carefully and gently. Follow the manufacturer's instructions carefully.

_____ Remove contact lenses. If the client wears contact lenses, they must be removed before starting the procedure.

_____ Client consultation. Discuss with the client the desired length of the lashes and the effect she hopes to achieve.

_____ Seat client. Place the client in the makeup chair with her head at a comfortable working height. The client's face should be well and evenly lit, but avoid shining the light directly into the eyes. Work from behind or to the side of the client. Avoid working directly in front of the client whenever possible.

Procedure

_____ Apply adhesive. Apply a thin strip of lash adhesive to the base of the lash and allow a few seconds for it to set.

_____ Prepare lashes. Brush the client's eyelashes to make sure they are clean and free of foreign matter, such as mascara particles. If the client's lashes are straight, they can be curled with an eyelash curler before you apply the artificial lashes.

_____ Carefully remove the eyelash band from the package.

_____ Feather lash. Feather the lash by nipping into it with the points of your scissors. This creates a more natural look.

_____ Apply the lower lash. Lower lash application is optional, as it tends to look more unnatural. Trim the lash as necessary and apply adhesive in the same way you did for the upper lash. Place the lash on top of the client's lower lash. Place the shorter lash toward the center of the eye and the longer lash toward the outer part of the lid.

_____ Shape eyelash. Start with the upper lash. If it is too long to fit the curve of the upper eyelid, trim the outside edge. Use your fingers to bend the lash into a horseshoe shape to make it more flexible so it fits the contour of the eyelid.

23

6

ESSENTIAL EXPERIENCE *continued*

_____ Apply the lash. Start with the shorter part of the lash and place it on the inner corner of the eye, toward the nose. Position the rest of the artificial lash as close to the client's own lash as possible. Use the rounded end of a lash liner brush or tweezers to press the lash on. Be very careful and gentle when applying the lashes. If eyeliner is to be used, the line is usually drawn on the eyelid before the lash is applied and retouched when the artificial lash is in place.

Cleanup/Sanitation

_____ Sanitize your workstation.

_____ Wash your hands with soap and warm water.

_____ Disinfect implements such as the eyelash curler.

_____ Place all towels, linens, and makeup cape in a hamper.

_____ Clean and sanitize brushes using a commercial brush sanitizer.

_____ Discard all disposable items, such as sponges, pads, spatulas, and applicators.

ESSENTIAL RUBRICS

Rubrics are used in education for organizing and interpreting data gathered from observations of student performance. It is a clearly developed scoring document used to differentiate between levels of development in a specific skill performance or behavior. A rubric is provided in this study guide as a self-assessment tool to aid you in your behavior development.

Rate your performance according to the following scale:

(1) Development Opportunity: There is little or no evidence of competency; Assistance is needed; Performance includes multiple errors.

(2) Fundamental: There is beginning evidence of competency; Task is completed alone; Performance includes few errors.

(3) Competent: There is detailed and consistent evidence of competency; Task is completed alone; Performance includes rare errors.

(4) Strength: There is detailed evidence of highly creative, inventive, mature presence of competency.

Space is provided for comments to assist you in improving your performance and achieving a higher rating.

PROFESSIONAL MAKEUP APPLICATION PROCEDURE

Performance Assessed	1	2	3	4	Improvement Plan
Pre-service sanitation and set up completed					
Performed client consultation					
Washed and sanitized hands					
Properly draped client					
Applied cleansing cream					
Removed cleanser residue					
Applied astringent or toner					
Applied moisturizer if applicable					
Groomed eyebrows					
Applied foundation					
Applied concealer					
Applied powder					
Applied eye color					
Applied eyeliner					
Applied eyebrow color					
Applied cheek color					
Applied lip color					
Post-service cleanup and appointment scheduling completed					

23

ESSENTIAL RUBRICS—CONT'D

BAND LASHES APPLICATION PROCEDURE

Performance Assessed	1	2	3	4	Improvement Plan
Pre-service sanitation and set up completed					
Performed client consultation					
Washed and sanitized hands					
Properly prepared and draped client					
Removed eye makeup					
Brushed natural eyelashes					
Removed eyelash band from package					
Trimmed eyelash band to fit eye					
Feathered lash if needed					
Applied thin strip of lash adhesive					
Applied the upper band lashes					
Applied lower lash if desired					
Proceeded with additional services as desired					
Post-service cleanup and appointment scheduling completed					

ESSENTIAL REVIEW

Using the following words, fill in the blanks below to form a thorough review of Chapter 23: Facial Makeup. Words or terms may be used more than once or not at all.

antiseptic	discolorations	lighter	straight
bleeding	double-dip	lip	strip
blend	eye tabbing	matte	thicker
blues	eyeliner	paraffin	widening
cheek color	face powder	paste-like	yellow
complementary	foundation	pink	yellow or gold
concealers	frame	powder foundation	
contour	high arch	shape	
cream	inner rim	smooth	

1. Affixing individual eyelashes to a client is referred to as _____ .

2. A cosmetic, usually tinted, that is used as a base or as a protective film applied before powder is known as _____ .

3. _____ foundation, also known as oil-based, is a considerably thicker product, often sold in a jar or a tin and may or may not contain water.

4. Mineral _____ is applied with a large fluffy brush and contains a lot of pigment for coverage.

5. _____ are available in tins, jars, and tubes with wands in a range of colors to coordinate with or match natural skin tones.

6. _____ is a cosmetic powder, sometimes tinted or scented, that is used to add a matte or non-shiny finish to the face.

7. _____ gives a natural-looking glow to the cheeks, but can also be used to add a little color to the face.

8. When applying cheek color, _____ outward and upward toward the temples.

9. Lip color is a cosmetic in a _____ form, usually in a metal or plastic tube, manufactured in a wide range of colors.

ESSENTIAL REVIEW *continued*

10. In addition to outlining the lips, lip liner helps to keep lip color from _____ into the small lines around the mouth.

11. Eye shadows are applied on the eyelids to accentuate or contour them and come in a variety of finishes, including metallic, _____ , frost, shimmer, and dewy.

12. A highlight color is _____ than the client's skin tone and may have any finish, including matte or iridescent.

13. A _____ color is deeper and darker than the client's skin tone and is applied to minimize a specific area to create contour.

14. The cosmetic used to outline and emphasize the eyes is called _____ .

15. Eyeliner pencils consist of a _____ wax or hardened oil base with a variety of additives to create color.

16. According to the American Medical Association, eye pencils should not be used to color the _____ of the eyes.

17. Eyebrow pencils or shadows are used to darken eyebrows, to fill in sparse areas, or to _____ the eyebrows.

18. Mascara is used to enhance the natural lashes making them appear _____ and longer.

19. Warm colors are dominated by _____ tones.

20. Cool colors suggest coolness and are dominated by _____ .

21. When choosing eye makeup colors, consider contrasting eye color with _____ colors to emphasize the eye color most effectively.

22. When choosing makeup colors, take care to coordinate cheek and _____ colors within the same color family.

23. When applying mascara to a client, use a disposable mascara wand and dip into a clean tube of mascara, taking care to never _____ .

ESSENTIAL REVIEW *continued*

24. If eyes are close-set, they can be made to appear farther apart by
_____ the distance between the eyebrows and extending
them outward slightly.

25. When arching brows for a long face, making them almost
_____ can create the illusion of a shorter face.

26. A square face will appear more oval if there is a _____ on the
ends of the eyebrows.

27. For ruddy skin, apply a _____ or green foundation to affected
areas, blending carefully.

28. For sallow skin, apply a _____ or violet-based foundation on
the affected areas and blend carefully into the jaw and neck.

29. Band lashes are also called _____ lashes.

30. As a safety precaution when giving a facial, keep fingernails
_____ and avoid scratching the client's skin.

ESSENTIAL DISCOVERIES AND ACCOMPLISHMENTS

In the space below, jot some notes about what concepts of this chapter were hardest for you to understand or remember. Imagine finding yourself suddenly in the role of "teacher" and consider what you would tell your "students" about these difficult concepts. Share your Essential Discoveries with some of the other students in your class and ask if they are helpful to them. You may want to revise your notes based on good ideas shared by your peers. Under Accomplishments, list at least three things you have accomplished since your last entry that relate to your career goals.

Discoveries:

_____

_____

_____

_____

_____

_____

_____

_____

_____

_____

Accomplishments:

_____

_____

_____

_____

_____

NAIL DISEASES & DISORDERS

A Motivating Moment: "The way I see it, if you want the rainbow, you gotta put up with the rain."—Dolly Parton

ESSENTIAL OBJECTIVES

After studying this chapter and completing the Essential Companion components, you should be able to:

1. List and describe the various disorders and irregularities of nails.

2. Recognize diseases of the nails that should not be treated in the salon.

ESSENTIAL NAIL STRUCTURE AND GROWTH

I want to be a hairstylist, not a scientist or doctor; why do I need to learn about nail diseases and disorders?

Nail disorders and diseases are certainly not the most glamorous portion of your training in cosmetology, but could be one of the most essential. More infections are spread through the nails and hands than any other area of the body. You actually have a greater chance of contracting a nail disease from a client than a skin disease or head lice. Therefore, careful analysis of the client's hands and nails is essential both to your safety and that of your clients. Think about it. If you contract an infection, it may prevent you from working for an extended period of time and that will cost you money, both in lost income and medical expenses. So, learning about the diseases and disorders associated with nails is extremely relevant to your future success and well-being.

ESSENTIAL CONCEPTS

What do I need to know about nail diseases and disorders in order to provide quality manicuring and pedicuring services?

You will need to be able to discern between a disorder and an infectious disease, which must be referred to a physician for treatment. When you've gained that knowledge, you can proceed confidently with appropriate nail services knowing that you and your client are not at risk. Refer to Chapter 8 for more information on the structure and growth of the nail.

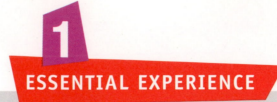

ESSENTIAL EXPERIENCE

Windowpane

Windowpaning is the process of transferring key elements, points, or steps in a lesson into visual images that are hand sketched into the squares or "panes" of a matrix. Let your mind think in pictures and sketch the essential concepts printed in each of the following windowpanes. Don't be concerned with your artistic ability. Use lines and stick figures to depict the concepts requested for the various conditions of the nail.

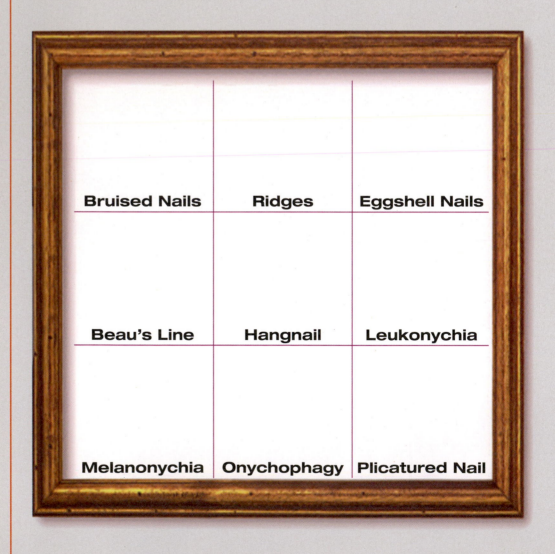

Bruised Nails	Ridges	Eggshell Nails
Beau's Line	Hangnail	Leukonychia
Melanonychia	Onychophagy	Plicatured Nail

2

ESSENTIAL EXPERIENCE

Nail Disorders, Irregularities, and Diseases

Label each of the following pictures or illustrations using the terms below. Use your standard textbook and other references in the school's library to assist you.

Eggshell nail
Beau's lines
Hangnail
Leukonychia spots
Melanonychia
Onychophagy

Onychorrhexis
Plicatured nail
Onychocryptosis
Onycholysis
Onychomadesis
Nail psoriasis

Paronychia
Pyogenic granuloma
Tinea pedis
Onychomycosis

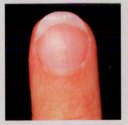 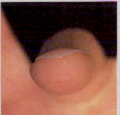 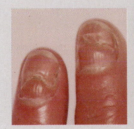 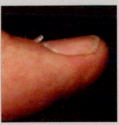

_____   _____   _____   _____

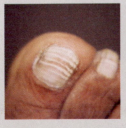 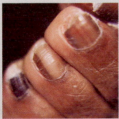 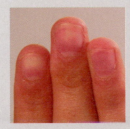 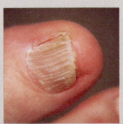

_____   _____   _____   _____

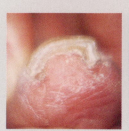
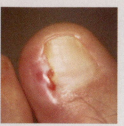
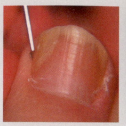
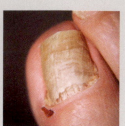

_____   _____   _____   _____

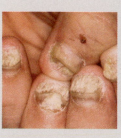
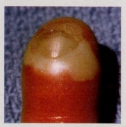
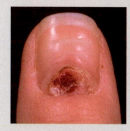
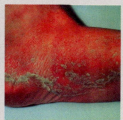

_____   _____   _____   _____

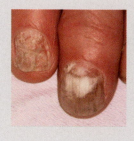

_____

3

Matching Exercise—Technical Terms Versus Common Terms

Match the following essential terms with their respective common term or identifying phrase.

_____ Bruised nail

_____ Melanonychia

_____ Leukonychia

_____ Nail psoriasis

_____ Onychomycosis

_____ Pterygium

_____ Onychophagy

_____ Onychorrhexis

_____ Hangnail

_____ Eggshell

_____ Onychosis

_____ Tinea pedis

_____ Paronychia

_____ Onychia

_____ Onychocryptosis

_____ Pyogenic granuloma

1. Bitten nails.

2. Living skin splits around nail.

3. Surface of nail plate appears rough and pitted.

4. Blood clot under nail plate.

5. White spots.

6. Fungal infection.

7. Darkening of fingernails or toenails.

8. Noticeably thin, white nail plates; more flexible than normal nails.

9. Any deformity or disease of the nails.

10. Inflammation of surrounding tissues.

11. Fungal infections of the feet.

12. Ingrown nails.

13. Severe inflammation of the nail in which a lump of red tissue grows up from nail bed to nail plate.

14. Skin is stretched by the nail plate.

15. Split or brittle nails.

16. Inflammation of matrix with formation of pus and shedding of the nail.

24

4

ESSENTIAL EXPERIENCE

Word Search

After identifying the appropriate word from the clues listed below, locate the word in the following word search puzzle.

Word	Clue
_____	Fungal infection of the feet.
_____	Dark purplish spots due to injury.
_____	Folded nail.
_____	Run vertically down the length of natural nail.
_____	Thin, white nail plate and more flexible than normal nails.
_____	May cause infections of the feet and hands.
_____	White spots in the nail.
_____	Split or brittle nails.
_____	Darkening of the fingernails or toenails.
_____	Visible depressions across the width of the nail plate.
_____	Bitten nails.

```
A G E T I N E A P E D I S J P C F U
L R L N P H I Y Z H V V H K Z E N I
G X E F I L Y D M N I K N S B G J S
C Y U O X L I G J Z I B C L B Z E N
T D K I F L S C Y K R H Q E H G E X
P Z O Z R A T U A N B T A C D G M Z
A J N C X F Q S A T U M D I G K P X
I L Y Y O A C H Y E U Z R S Z Q H K
H I C G C T J X Y W B R H V U H X W
C A H A F Y A B G H E E E S U U A U
Y N I H A V J M R D L C F D R H I U
N D A P N V T H D L Q W K U N R J R
O E T O J D H S N U Z F B J N A Y R
N S N H B C P A D B E F P O Z G I P
A I C C K K I O P Z G B W O B H I L
L U Z Y K L P R X N U U D T U A D V
E R T N S X J U J E J V S Y K K K Z
M B V O C S I X E H R R O H C Y N O
```

Word Search

After identifying the appropriate word from the clues listed below, locate the word in the following word search puzzle.

Word	Clue
_____	Separation or falling off of a nail plate.
_____	Deformity or disease of the nail.
_____	Lifting of the nail plate.
_____	Severe inflammation of the nail.
_____	Inflammation of the nail matrix.
_____	Ingrown nails.
_____	Bacterial inflammation of surrounding tissue of the nail.
_____	Tiny pits or severe roughness.
_____	A fungal infection of the nail plate.

```
O O O L D V Y A I H C Y N O R A P A
I N N O M L C G C M D Y Z B P W M H
E W Y Y K S X B L M W L D U J O A V
P F T C C Y B G X H O W D U L J P J
S S Y O H H I R S L U Y M U C A J F
I B K H Q O I G T G Z Y N R V S Q S
S O N H H I C A Q R Q A M S C U V I
O M D K U E R R L K R H P G Q T S S
C R X Q H P P V Y G P L S D Q O I E
Y N E Q D D Z N C P K M K J J S S D
M Z W W V L U I Q G T V B X T I Y A
O E J I K H N K D P O O J J I S L M
H I L C G E X V I A C F S C D O O O
C W S K G W M B W J A F X I K H H H
Y L J O O H K Z S B Z C Y R S C C C
N W Y C A U W A L F W Z D U W Y Y Y
O P R L F L Z D B C I U N Z M N N N
N A I L P S O R I A S I S X O O O O
```

ESSENTIAL EXPERIENCE

Technical Term Mnemonics

Mnemonics are aids that can be used to assist your memory. They can be words or phrase associations, songs, or any other method that will trigger in your memory key terms or information contained in a lesson. For example, if you were trying to remember the three primary areas of haircutting, **b**lunt, **g**raduated, and **l**ayered, you might make up a sentence using the first letter of each type of haircutting. In this case, the mnemonic might be **B**renda **G**ot **L**ost. Using this learning tool, try to develop a mnemonic for each of the following technical terms in the study of the nail. For example: Ony**chop**tosis is the periodic shedding or falling off of the nail. Within the technical term is the word "chop." You might relate the word "chop" to the chopping off or falling of the nail and remember the meaning of onychoptosis. Give it a try with the other terms. Don't limit yourself to words. You can draw pictures or visualize circumstances that will cause you to remember the technical term.

1. Beau's line
_____
_____

2. Leukonychia spots
_____
_____

3. Melanonychia
_____
_____

4. Onychophagy
_____
_____

5. Onychorrhexis
_____
_____

6. Plicatured nail
_____
_____

7. Pterygium
_____
_____

8. Onychosis
_____
_____

9. Onychia
_____
_____

10. Onychocryptosis
_____
_____

11. Onycholysis
_____
_____

12. Onychomadesis
_____
_____

13. Psoriasis
_____
_____

14. Paronychia
_____
_____

15. Onychomycosis
_____
_____

ESSENTIAL REVIEW

Complete the following review of Chapter 24: Nail Diseases and Disorders, by circling the correct answer to each question.

1. A healthy nail appears slightly _____ in color.
   a) yellow
   b) pink
   c) blue
   d) purple

2. _____ are caused by uneven growth of the nails.
   a) furrows
   b) depressions
   c) ridges
   d) pterygium

3. _____ on the nails are known as leukonychia.
   a) white spots
   b) blue spots
   c) white stripes
   d) vertical ridges

4. Bitten nails, a result of an acquired nervous habit, are known as _____ .
   a) onychauxis
   b) onychatrophia
   c) onychophagy
   d) pterygium

5. An abnormal condition that occurs when skin is stretched by the nail plate.
   a) onychauxis
   b) onychatrophia
   c) onychophagy
   d) pterygium

6. Hangnails are treated by _____ .
   a) hot oil manicures
   b) filing straight across
   c) avoiding polish use
   d) firm use of metal pusher

7. A parasite, which under some circumstances may cause infections of the feet and hands, is _____ .
   a) flagella
   b) fungi
   c) mold
   d) fungus

8. Darkening of the fingernails or toenails is technically known as _____ .
   a) melanonychia
   b) leukonychia
   c) onychatrophia
   d) onychauxis

ESSENTIAL REVIEW   *continued*

9. Onychocryptosis is the technical term for _____ .
   a) split nails
   b) bitten nails
   c) bruised nails
   d) ingrown nails

10. A fungal infection of the nail plate is _____ .
    a) onychauxis
    b) onychatrophia
    c) onychophagy
    d) onychomycosis

11. An infectious and inflammatory condition of the tissues surrounding the nails is known as _____ .
    a) onychia
    b) onychomycosis
    c) paronychia
    d) onychocryptosis

12. The technical term for loosening of the nail without shedding or falling off is _____ .

    a) onycholysis
    b) onychogryposis
    c) onychomycosis
    d) onychophosis

13. A growth of horny epithelium in the nail bed is known as _____ .
    a) onycholysis
    b) onychogryposis
    c) onychophyma
    d) onychophosis

14. A condition in which a blood clot forms under the nail plate is known as _____ .

    a) hangnail
    b) bruised nail
    c) eggshell nail
    d) plicatured nail

15. A condition which affects the surface of the natural nail plate, causing it to appear rough and pitted, is known as _____ .
    a) nail pterygium
    b) plicatured nail
    c) nail psoriasis
    d) pincer nails

ESSENTIAL DISCOVERIES AND ACCOMPLISHMENTS

In the space below, jot some notes about what concepts of this chapter were hardest for you to understand or remember. Imagine finding yourself suddenly in the role of "teacher" and consider what you would tell your "students" about these difficult concepts. Share your Essential Discoveries with some of the other students in your class and ask if they are helpful to them. You may want to revise your notes based on good ideas shared by your peers. Under Accomplishments, list at least three things you have accomplished since your last entry that relate to your career goals.

Discoveries:

_____

_____

_____

_____

_____

_____

_____

_____

_____

Accomplishments:

_____

_____

_____

_____

MANICURING & PEDICURING

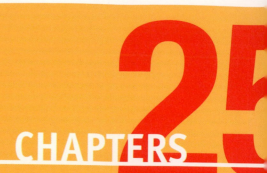

This chapter contains information and activities related to both Chapters 25 and 26 of *Milady's Standard Cosmetology,* 2008 edition.

A Motivating Moment: *"An optimist is a person who sees a green light everywhere. The pessimist sees only the red light. But the truly wise person is color blind."—Dr. Albert Schweitzer*

ESSENTIAL OBJECTIVES

After studying this chapter and completing the Essential Companion components, you should be able to:

1. Identify the four types of nail implements and/or tools required to perform a manicure.

2. Demonstrate the safe and correct handling of nail implements and tools.

3. Exhibit a proper setup of a manicuring table.

4. Demonstrate the necessary three-part procedure requirements for nail services.

5. Identify the five basic nail shapes.

6. Perform a basic and conditioning oil manicure incorporating all safety, sanitation, and disinfection requirements.

ESSENTIAL OBJECTIVES *continued*

7. Demonstrate the correct technique for the application of nail polish.

8. Perform the five basic nail polish applications.

9. Perform the hand and arm massage movements associated with manicuring.

10. Perform a paraffin wax hand treatment.

11. Display all sanitation, disinfection, and safety requirements essential to nail and hand care services.

12. Define and understand aromatherapy.

13. Identify carrier oils and understand their use.

14. Understand how aromatherapy can be incorporated into a service.

15. Identify and explain the equipment and materials needed for a pedicure.

16. List the steps in the procedures and precautions for a pedicure.

17. Demonstrate the proper procedures and precautions for a pedicure.

18. Describe the proper technique to use in filing toenails.

19. Describe the proper technique for trimming the nails.

20. Demonstrate your ability to perform foot massage properly.

21. Understand proper cleaning and disinfecting of pedicure equipment.

ESSENTIAL MANICURING AND PEDICURING

Why are manicuring and pedicuring so important in my career as a cosmetologist?

It may help to understand a little of the history of manicuring in order to understand its relevance in today's society. The word manicure comes from the Latin word *manus* (which means hand) and the word *cura* (which means care). So, manicuring means just that, to improve the appearance of the hands and nails. You need to be able to provide this important service to your clients, but you also must maintain your own hands and nails in the best possible condition. After all, you will be touching your clients with your hands during every service you offer. It is important that your nails are smooth and don't scratch the client's skin or scalp.

The early societies of Egypt and China considered long, polished, and colored fingernails as a mark of distinction between the commoners and the aristocrats. Nails were shaped with pumice stones and colored with vegetable dyes. In the late 1800s, painted fingernails became a trend among the elite in Paris. Manicuring as a service and wearing nail polish became so popular in the 1920s that barber shops began to offer services for nails to both men and women. By the late 1950s, most states began to require licensure for this special service.

What do I need to know about manicuring and pedicuring in order to provide a quality service?

As with other services you provide you will need to thoroughly consult with each client to learn what his or her specific desires are with the nail service. You will need to be able to file and shape the nails to the desired shape. You must be able to gather and properly use all the implements and equipment required in the various nail procedures. You will learn the importance of being able to provide an effective hand and arm or foot massage in manicuring and pedicuring.

1

Windowpane—Nail Shapes

Windowpaning is the process of transferring key elements, points, or steps in a lesson into visual images that are hand sketched into the squares or "panes" of a matrix. Let your mind think in pictures and sketch the essential concepts printed in each of the following windowpanes. Don't be concerned with your artistic ability. Use lines and stick figures to depict the concepts requested.

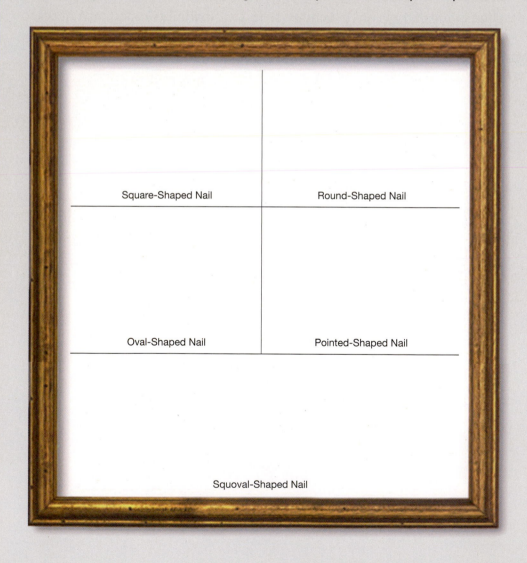

Square-Shaped Nail	Round-Shaped Nail
Oval-Shaped Nail	Pointed-Shaped Nail
Squoval-Shaped Nail	

ESSENTIAL EXPERIENCE

Implements

Identify each of the manicuring implements depicted below.

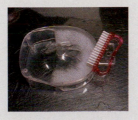

_____

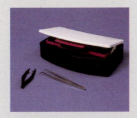

_____

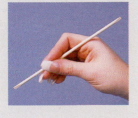

_____

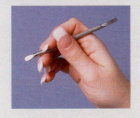

_____

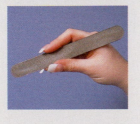

_____

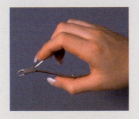

_____

3 ESSENTIAL EXPERIENCE

Matching Exercise

Match the following essential terms with their identifying phrases or definition.

_____ Carrier oil

_____ Chamois buffer

_____ Mild abrasives

_____ Pledgets

_____ Pumice powder

_____ Supply tray

_____ Wooden pusher

_____ Tweezers

_____ Nail brush

_____ Nail clippers

1. Used to add shine to the nail and smooth wavy ridges.

2. Holds cosmetics.

3. Used to lift small bits of debris from nail plate.

4. Used to clean fingernails.

5. Used to shorten the nail plate.

6. Used to remove cuticle tissue from nail plate.

7. A base oil in aromatherapy.

8. Used to smooth nails and skin.

9. Fiber-free cotton squares.

10. Abrasive derived from volcanic rock.

4

Manicure Table Setup

Identify the parts, tools, and implements found in the manicure table setup shown below. Reminder: The table setup recommended by your instructor is equally correct.

1. Towel-wrapped cushion.

2. Bowl of warm, soapy water to left of client.

3. Disinfected metal implements and a new orangewood stick on towel.

4. Cream, lotions, and polishes in order to be used, placed to left of technician.

5. Disinfected abrasive and fresh emery boards to right of technician.

6. Small plastic bag attached to table, either on right or left, for waste materials.

7. Fresh disinfectant solution for implements.

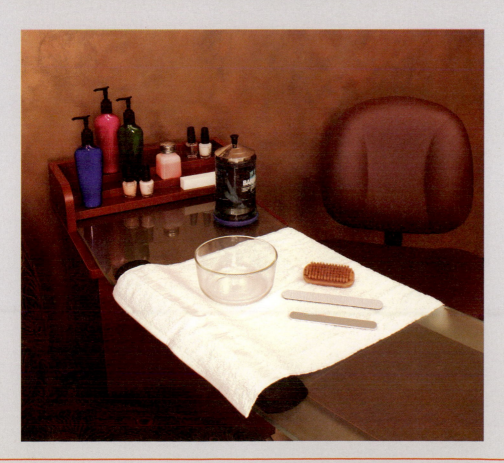

5

ESSENTIAL EXPERIENCE

Word Scramble

Scramble	Correct Word
alin life	_ _ _ _ _ _ _ _
	Clue: Used for shaping and smoothing the free edge
litucce presinp	_ _ _ _ _ _ _ _ _ _ _ _ _ _
	Clue: Used for trimming the cuticle
lian fubref	_ _ _ _ _ _ _ _ _ _
	Clue: Used for buffing and polishing the nail
rengfi wblo	_ _ _ _ _ _ _ _ _ _
	Clue: Holds warm, soapy water
tuclice hspure	_ _ _ _ _ _ _ _ _ _ _ _ _
	Clue: Loosens and pushes back the cuticle
cirtleec retahe	_ _ _ _ _ _ _ _ _ _ _ _ _ _
	Clue: Heats oil
ailn sbruh	_ _ _ _ _ _ _ _ _ _
	Clue: Used for cleansing nails and fingertips
yulpps ytar	_ _ _ _ _ _ _ _ _ _ _
	Clue: Holds cosmetics for the nails
ezsewret	_ _ _ _ _ _ _ _ _
	Clue: Used for lifting small bits of cuticle
rnienaotc	_ _ _ _ _ _ _ _ _
	Clue: Holds clean absorbent cotton

6

Manicure Table Setup Procedure

Put the following steps for setting up the table for a manicure in the proper order.

_____ Prepare for waste disposal.

_____ Place abrasives.

_____ Place fingerbowl.

_____ Prepare arm cushion.

_____ Place polishes.

_____ Prepare drawer.

_____ Fill disinfectant container.

_____ Clean table.

_____ Place products.

7 ESSENTIAL EXPERIENCE

Manicure Procedure

Put the following steps for a plain manicure in the appropriate order.

____ Apply polish.

____ Dry hand.

____ Bleach nails (optional).

____ Repeat steps 5–9 on other hand.

____ Loosen and remove cuticles.

____ Apply nail oil.

____ Bevel nails.

____ Clean nails.

____ Choose a color.

____ Clean under free edge.

____ Apply cuticle remover.

____ Buff with high-shine buffer.

____ Apply lotion and massage.

____ Remove old polish.

____ Remove traces of oil.

____ Shape nails.

____ Soften cuticle.

____ Clip away dead tags of skin.

8 ESSENTIAL EXPERIENCE

Partners for Pedicure

Choose a partner and provide a pedicure service to each other. Rate each other's procedure according to the following evaluation form. Circle the numeric score you would assign the service you just received, using the following rating scale.

1 = Poor;   2 = Below Average;   3 = Average;   4 = Good;   5 = Excellent

1 2 3 4 5   **1.** You were seated comfortably and asked to remove shoes and socks or stockings.

1 2 3 4 5   **2.** All required equipment, implements, and materials were arranged.

1 2 3 4 5   **3.** Your feet were placed on clean paper towels on a footrest.

1 2 3 4 5   **4.** Nail technician's hands were washed and sanitized.

1 2 3 4 5   **5.** Two basins were filled with warm water to cover ankles.

1 2 3 4 5   **6.** Antiseptic or antibacterial soap was added to one basin; both feet were placed in bath for 3 to 5 minutes.

1 2 3 4 5   **7.** Feet were removed, rinsed, and wiped dry.

1 2 3 4 5   **8.** Old polish was thoroughly removed from nails of both feet.

1 2 3 4 5   **9.** Toenails of left foot were clipped.

1 2 3 4 5   **10.** Toe separators were inserted.

1 2 3 4 5   **11.** Toenails were filed straight across, rounding them slightly at the corners to conform to the shape of the toes.

1 2 3 4 5   **12.** Foot file was used on ball and heel of left foot to remove dry skin and smooth down callus growth.

1 2 3 4 5   **13.** Toe separator was removed and left foot was placed in warm, soapy water.

1 2 3 4 5   **14.** Steps 9–13 were completed on the right foot.

1 2 3 4 5   **15.** Left foot was removed from basin, rinsed, dried, and toe separators were inserted.

1 2 3 4 5   **16.** Cuticle solvent was applied under free edge of each toenail of left foot with cotton-tipped orangewood stick.

1 2 3 4 5   **17.** Cuticle was gently loosened with the cotton-tipped orangewood stick. Cuticle was kept moist with additional lotion or water. Excessive pressure was not used. Cuticle was not cut.

1 2 3 4 5   **18.** Left foot was rinsed and dried.

1 2 3 4 5   **19.** Cream or lotions were applied.

1 2 3 4 5   **20.** Left foot was massaged and placed on a clean towel on floor.

1 2 3 4 5   **21.** Steps 15–20 were repeated on the right foot.

1 2 3 4 5   **22.** Lotion or cream was removed from toenails.

1 2 3 4 5   **23.** Base coat, two color coats, and top coat were applied.

1 2 3 4 5   **24.** Post-service steps were completed.

25 & 26

ESSENTIAL RUBRICS

Rubrics are used in education for organizing and interpreting data gathered from observations of student performance. It is a clearly developed scoring document used to differentiate between levels of development in a specific skill performance or behavior. A rubric is provided in this study guide as a self-assessment tool to aid you in your behavior development.

Rate your performance according to the following scale:

(1) Development Opportunity: There is little or no evidence of competency; Assistance is needed; Performance includes multiple errors.

(2) Fundamental: There is beginning evidence of competency; Task is completed alone; Performance includes few errors.

(3) Competent: There is detailed and consistent evidence of competency; Task is completed alone; Performance includes rare errors.

(4) Strength: There is detailed evidence of highly creative, inventive, mature presence of competency.

Space is provided for comments to assist you in improving your performance and achieving a higher rating.

MANICURE TABLE PREPARATION PROCEDURE

Performance Assessed	1	2	3	4	Improvement Plan
Cleaned table with disinfectant solution					
Prepared arm cushion					
Filled disinfectant container					
Placed products					
Placed abrasives					
Placed fingerbowl and brush					
Prepared for waste disposal					
Placed polishes					
Prepared drawer					

PRE-SERVICE PROCEDURE

Performance Assessed	1	2	3	4	Improvement Plan
Sanitized implements					
Rinsed implements and dried thoroughly					
Immersed implements					
Washed hands					
Rinsed and dried implements					
Followed approve storage procedure					

POST-SERVICE PROCEDURE

Performance Assessed	1	2	3	4	Improvement Plan
Scheduled next appointment					
Advised client on home maintenance					
Promoted product sales					
Cleaned work area					
Disinfected implements					
Recorded service information					

ESSENTIAL RUBRICS—CONT'D

HAND MASSAGE PROCEDURE

Performance Assessed	1	2	3	4	Improvement Plan
Pre-service sanitation and set up completed					
Applied massage lotion					
Relaxer movement					
Joint movement on fingers					
Circular movement in palm					
Circular movement on wrist					
Circular movement on back of hands and fingers					
Effleurage on arms					
Wringing/friction movement					
Kneading movement					
Rotation on elbow					
Proceed with other services as desired					
Post-service cleanup and appointment scheduling completed					

PLAIN MANICURE PROCEDURE

Performance Assessed	1	2	3	4	Improvement Plan
Pre-service sanitation and set up completed					
Performed client consultation					
Washing and sanitized hands					
Removed polish					
Shaped the nails					
Softened cuticles					
Cleaned nails					
Dried hands					
Applied cuticle remover					
Loosened and removed cuticles					
Nipped dead skin tags					
Cleaned under free edge					
Repeated on opposite hand					
Bleached nails (optional)					
Buffed nails with high shine buffer					
Applied nail oil					
Beveled nails					
Applied lotion and massaged					
Removed traces of oil					
Selected polish color and applied					
Post-service cleanup and appointment scheduling completed					

25 & 26

ESSENTIAL RUBRICS—CONT'D

BASIC PEDICURE PROCEDURE

Performance Assessed	1	2	3	4	Improvement Plan
Pre-service sanitation and set up completed					
Performed client consultation					
Washed and sanitized hands					
Removed shoes and socks					
Soaked feet					
Dried feet thoroughly					
Removed existing polish					
Clipped nails					
Filed nails					
Used foot file					
Rinsed foot; placed other foot in bath					
Repeated steps on other foot					
Brushed nails					
Applied cuticle remover					
Removed cuticle tissue					
Rinsed, brushed, and dried foot					
Applied lotion, cream or oil					
Massaged foot					
Repeated steps on other foot					
Removed traces of lotion					
Applied polish					
Post-service cleanup and appointment scheduling completed					

ESSENTIAL RUBRICS—CONT'D

FULL SERVICE PEDICURE PROCEDURE

Performance Assessed	1	2	3	4	Improvement Plan
Pre-service sanitation and set up completed					
Performed client consultation					
Washed and sanitized hands					
Soaked the feet					
Removed polish					
Applied cuticle remover					
Used curette					
Trimmed toenails					
Removed cuticle tissue					
Smoothed edges of nail plate					
Smoothed remainder of nail with abrasive file					
Repeated steps on other foot					
Exfoliated dry skin off feet					
Smoothed calluses					
Rinsed					
Applied masque					
Scrubbed and treated calluses on other foot					
Completed foot and leg massage					
Applied polish if desired					
Post-service cleanup and appointment scheduling completed					

25 & 26

ESSENTIAL REVIEW

Complete the following multiple choice test by circling the correct answer.

1. When you perform nail services, you use permanent tools called:
   a) equipment
   b) implements
   c) materials
   d) cosmetics

2. Disposable implements include:
   a) nail clippers
   b) metal pushers
   c) tweezers
   d) wooden pushers

3. In a manicure service, to shape the free edge you use a/an:
   a) wooden pusher
   b) metal pusher
   c) abrasive file
   d) tweezers

4. During a manicure procedure, if you draw blood, the implement should be:
   a) cleaned and disinfected
   b) rinsed with water
   c) bagged and discarded
   d) wiped off with cotton

5. The benefit of using nail clippers to shorten nail length is to:
   a) create high shine
   b) strengthen weak nails
   c) reduce filing time
   d) reduce splitting

6. To smooth out wavy ridges and create a high shine, use an:
   a) chamois buffer
   b) ridge filler
   c) abrasive file
   d) nail clipper

7. When you perform nail services, those supplies used during a service that must be replaced for each client are called:
   a) equipment
   b) implements
   c) materials
   d) cosmetics

8. Lamps attached to a manicure table should have a bulb of _____ watts.
   a) 25–30
   b) 30–35
   c) 40–60
   d) 60-75

9. After you use metal implements and before you place them in disinfectant, they must be:
   a) cleaned with a towel
   b) cleaned in autoclave
   c) rinsed in alcohol
   d) washed with soap and water

continued

10. An oil manicure is a recommended treatment for:
  a) flexible cuticles
  b) brittle nails
  c) short nails
  d) nail fungus

11. The implement used to clean fingernails and remove debris is called a:
  a) nail file
  b) nail brush
  c) wooden pusher
  d) chamois buffer

12. All non-disposable implements must be _____ in a disinfectant solution.
  a) quickly rinsed
  b) dipped slightly
  c) wiped thoroughly
  d) fully immersed

13. Removing nail cosmetics from their containers is accomplished with a
  a) wooden pusher
  b) plastic or metal spatula
  c) metal pusher
  d) cotton swab

14. Certain products such as alcohol, nail polish, nail monomers, and nail primers are considered to be:
  a) harmful
  b) sanitizers
  c) self-disinfecting
  d) strengtheners

15. As an added service in a manicure, a hand massage may be given before:
  a) polish
  b) pushing cuticles
  c) soaking fingers
  d) filing

16. After an oil manicure, before base coat is applied, you must:
  a) soak fingers in finger bowl
  b) remove all traces of oil
  c) apply cuticle remover
  d) wash hands thoroughly

17. When removing nail polish from nails with wrap resins, a/an _____ product is recommended.
  a) acetone
  b) oily
  c) non-acetone
  d) potassium

18. The best way to prevent excessive odors and control vapors from nail services in the salon is to use:
  a) plastic trash can
  b) ventilated receptacles with lids
  c) multiple paper bags
  d) metal receptacle with self-closing lid

19. Products designed to hasten the drying of nail polishes may be sprayed on or applied with a:
    a) wooden pusher
    b) cotton swab
    c) metal pusher
    d) dropper

20. One of the functions of a top coat or sealer is to make the nail polish:
    a) dry more quickly
    b) adhere to nail plate
    c) resistant to chipping
    d) appear thick and smooth

21. Nail hardeners include those with reinforcing fibers such as nylon, protein, and:
    a) potassium
    b) formaldehyde
    c) acetone
    d) UV gels

22. The base coat creates a colorless layer on the natural nail that improves:
    a) adhesion of polish
    b) and smoothes ridges
    c) discoloration and stains
    d) strength and rigidity

23. Another name for nail polish is:
    a) lotion
    b) cream
    c) lacquer
    d) oil

24. Yellow surface discoloration or stains on fingernails can be removed with:
    a) cuticle removers
    b) penetrating oils
    c) polish removers
    d) nail bleaches

25. Products used to soften dry skin around the nail plate and to increase the flexibility of natural nails are:
    a) cuticle removers
    b) penetrating oils
    c) polish removers
    d) nail bleaches

In the space below, jot some notes about what concepts of this chapter were hardest for you to understand or remember. Imagine finding yourself suddenly in the role of "teacher" and consider what you would tell your "students" about these difficult concepts. Share your Essential Discoveries with some of the other students in your class and ask if they are helpful to them. You may want to revise your notes based on good ideas shared by your peers. Under Accomplishments, list at least three things you have accomplished since your last entry that relate to your career goals.

Discoveries:

_____

_____

_____

_____

_____

_____

_____

_____

_____

Accomplishments:

_____

_____

_____

_____

25 & 26

ADVANCED NAIL TECHNIQUES

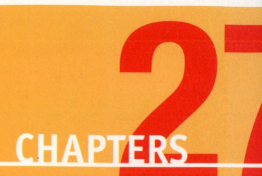

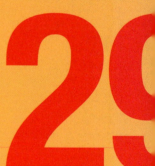

This chapter contains information and activities related to both Chapters 27, 28, and 29 of *Milady's Standard Cosmetology,* 2008 edition.

A Motivating Moment: "There are no evil thoughts except one: the refusal to think."—Ayn Rand

ESSENTIAL OBJECTIVES

After studying this chapter and completing the Essential Companion components, you should be able to:

1. Identify the supplies needed for nail tips and explain why they are needed.

2. Identify the three types of nail tips.

3. Demonstrate the proper procedure and precautions to use in applying nail tips.

4. Demonstrate the proper removal of tips.

5. List four kinds of nail wraps, and what they are used for.

6. Explain benefits of using silk, linen, fiberglass, and paper wraps.

7. Demonstrate the proper procedures and precautions to use in fabric wrap application.

ESSENTIAL OBJECTIVES   *continued*

8. Describe the maintenance of fabric wrap including a description of the 2-week and 4-week rebalance.

9. Explain how to use fabric wrap for crack repairs.

10. Demonstrate the proper procedure and precautions for fabric wrap removal.

11. Define no-light gels.

12. Demonstrate the proper procedures for applying no-light gels.

13. Explain acrylic (methacrylate) nail enhancement chemistry, and how it works.

14. List the supplies needed for acrylic nail enhancements application.

15. Demonstrate the proper procedures for applying acrylic nail enhancements, using forms over tips and on natural nails.

16. Practice safety precautions involving the application of nail primers.

17. Describe the proper procedure for maintaining healthy acrylic nail enhancements.

18. Perform regular rebalance procedures and repairs.

19. Implement the proper procedure for removal of acrylic nail enhancements.

20. Explain how the application of odorless acrylic products differs from the application of traditional acrylic products.

21. Describe the chemistry and main ingredients of UV gels.

22. Identify the supplies needed for UV gel application.

23. Demonstrate the proper procedures for maintaining UV gel services using forms, over tips, and on natural nails.

24. Describe the one-color and two-color method for applying UV gels.

25. Explain how to safely and correctly remove UV gels.

ESSENTIAL ADVANCED NAIL TECHNIQUES

Why do I need to learn about advanced nail techniques to be successful?

The nail industry experienced great expansion when the first acrylic artificial nail extensions were introduced in the early 1970s. The popular singer and actress Cher started a trend of very long nails which were squared off at the ends. By the 1980s, manufacturers had developed products which created very natural-looking artificial nails. It was then that the nail industry became the fastest growing area in the entire field of cosmetology and it continues to grow. Cosmetologists who fine-tune their skills with manicuring, pedicuring, and advanced nail techniques can earn a very good income.

ESSENTIAL CONCEPTS

What do I need to know about advanced nail techniques in order to provide a quality service?

You will need to become familiar and experienced with a variety of advanced nail techniques from nail tips and wraps to acrylic nail applications. It has been said that with today's technology, there is no reason for anyone who wants long beautiful nails not to have them. As a professional cosmetologist, you need to prepared to deliver those services that will meet that need.

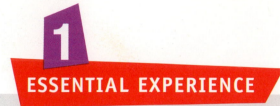

ESSENTIAL EXPERIENCE

Windowpane

Windowpaning is the process of transferring key elements, points, or steps in a lesson into visual images that are hand sketched into the squares or "panes" of a matrix. Let your mind think in pictures and sketch the essential concepts printed in each of the following windowpanes. Don't be concerned with your artistic ability. Use lines and stick figures to depict the concepts requested.

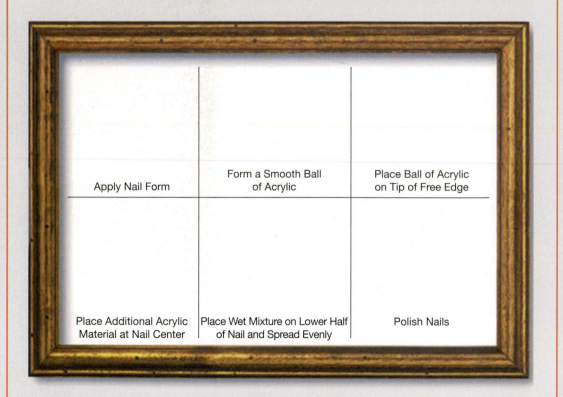

Apply Nail Form	Form a Smooth Ball of Acrylic	Place Ball of Acrylic on Tip of Free Edge
Place Additional Acrylic Material at Nail Center	Place Wet Mixture on Lower Half of Nail and Spread Evenly	Polish Nails

2

Pre- and Post-Service Procedures

Number the following steps for an advanced nail technique pre- and post-service procedure.

Nail Tip Pre-Service procedure

____ **Greet client.** Have client wash hands with soap and warm water. Thoroughly dry with fresh towel.

____ **Client consultation.** Complete card by recording responses and observations. Check for nail disorders, etc.

____ **Pre-service sanitation.**

____ **Standard table set-up.** Add abrasives, buffer blocks, nail adhesive, nail tips to table.

Nail Tip Post-Service Procedure

____ **Sanitation.** Clean and disinfect table, implements, and multi-use tools.

____ **Clean up area.** Cap glue and clean applicator tips in acetone.

____ **Sell retail products.** For home maintenance.

____ **Discard used materials.** Put in plastic bag and discard in a closed pail.

____ **Schedule appointment.** Follow-up or maintenance needed.

27-29

3

ESSENTIAL EXPERIENCE

Nail Tip Procedure

Nail Tip Application Procedure

_____ **Size tips.** Must completely cover nail plate from sidewall to sidewall and never more that one-third of the length of the nail plate. Tips should be pre-beveled along the cuticle edge. This reduces potential damage to natural nail. Place tips on towel in order of application.

_____ **Proceed with service.** Wraps, acrylics, or UV gels.

_____ **Trim nail tip.** To desired length with tip cutter or large nail clippers. Cut from one side, then the other. Cutting straight across weakens the plastic.

_____ **Apply dehydrator.** Use cotton-tipped wooden pusher or spray to apply dehydrator/cleanser to nails. It will remove more of the natural oil and dehydrate nail for better adhesion.

_____ **Remove polish.** Begin with client's left hand, little finger. Repeat on right hand.

_____ **Apply adhesive.** Place on nail plate to cover area where tip will be placed. Don't let run on skin; apply from middle of nail to free edge.

_____ **Slide on tips.** Stop, Rock, and Hold. Stop—find stop against free edge at 45°. Rock—rock tip on slowly. Hold—hold in place firmly for 5–10 seconds. If white spots or air bubbles, tip must be reapplied. (Also used for well-less tips.)

_____ **Shape nail.** Use abrasive to shape new, longer nail.

_____ **Buff nail/remove shine.** Buff lightly over nail plate with medium/fine (180 grit or higher) abrasive to remove natural oil. Remove the dust with nail brush.

_____ **Push back eponychium.** Use cotton-tipped orangewood stick to gently push back cuticle. Use light touch because cuticle is dry; no solvent.

_____ **Remove cuticle tissue.** Use cuticle remover and a wooden or metal pusher/curette. Carefully remove cuticle tissue from nail plate.

_____ **Finish blending.** Sand the shine off tip with medium to fine grit buff block file. Hold file flat. Holding at an angle can make a groove in nail plate.

4 ESSENTIAL EXPERIENCE

Word Scramble

Scramble	Correct Word
aosylrev	_ _ _ _ _ _ _ _

Clue: Any wraps, acrylic, or gel applied over the entire natural nail plate or tip.

erirmp	_ _ _ _ _ _

Clue: Substance that improves adhesion, or attachment, and prepares the nail surface for bonding with the acrylic material.

ernmoom	_ _ _ _ _ _ _

Clue: Substance made up of many small molecules that are not attached to one another.

irnguc	_ _ _ _ _ _

Clue: Hardening process that occurs when powdered and liquid acrylic are combined to form nails.

istp	_ _ _ _

Clue: Pre-formed artificial nails applied to the tips of the natural nails.

mryeolp	_ _ _ _ _ _ _

Clue: Hard substance formed by combining many small molecules, usually in a long chain-like structure.

nagricnlabe	_ _ _ _ _ _ _ _ _ _ _

Clue: Redefining the shape of the acrylic nail during a fill procedure.

sciracly	_ _ _ _ _ _ _ _

Clue: Sculptured nails; artificial nails created by combining a liquid acrylic product with a powdered product to form a soft ball that can easily be molded into a nail shape.

4

ESSENTIAL EXPERIENCE *continued*

slge

_ _ _ _

Clue: Strong, durable artificial nails that are brushed on the nail plate.

spwar

_ _ _ _ _ _

Clue: Corrective treatments that form a protective coating for damaged or fragile nails.

ytaasltc

_ _ _ _ _ _ _ _

Clue: Any substance having the power to increase the velocity of a chemical reaction.

ESSENTIAL EXPERIENCE

Word Search

After determining the correct words from the clues provided, locate the words in the word search puzzle.

Word	Clue
_____	Sculptured nails.
_____	Acrylic nails applied directly to the natural nail surface or nail tip.
_____	Hardening process for acrylic nails.
_____	Gel nail that hardens when exposed to a special light source, either ultraviolet or halogen.
_____	Substance made from many small molecules that are not attached to each other.
_____	Corrective treatment that forms a protective coating for damaged or fragile nails.
_____	Gel nail that hardens when an activator or accelerator is sprayed or brushed on.
_____	Any wrap, acrylic, or gel applied over the entire natural nail plate.
_____	Hard substance formed by combining many small molecules, usually in a long chain-like structure.
_____	Point where the nail plate meets the tip before it is glued to the nail.
_____	Substance that improves adhesion and prepares surface for bonding.
_____	Redefining the shape of acrylic nails during a fill procedure.

5

ESSENTIAL EXPERIENCE *continued*

```
A C R Y L I C N A I L S R Q X M Q Z
D S V B J N P O T S N O I T I S O P
I R Y P G F X L C E L U M B C E H P
N E N A Y T R G H U U M O G I I R M
N B O S L A Z Y I D P U W A P I O G
W A L H U R L A D E F J C V M N L E
G L I P Q B E R Y B D H A E O E S O
N A G E D B J V E T B N R M G P I S
I N H T E Z Q D O V R E E D P U A F
P C T J N R S L I C O R E K M A C E
P I G W K I C C O R I R W I T Q M N
A N E M L E U N Q P U L C L K T Y A
R G L P R H X R O C P Y Y U P G O N
W N Q Z W I H L T W J J K R R E A D
L L K U U C Y H M Z C Q T D C I Q C
I H L Y L M G M X U B G D X A A N N
A O T P E I N P H D L Q W Y M V Y G
N T O R L Z Q Y X K T Z S J G S M B
```

6

Client Consultation

Develop several open-ended questions that you would use in a client consultation prior to an advanced nail technique service and write them in the space provided.

1. _____
   _____

2. _____
   _____
   _____

3. _____
   _____

4. _____
   _____

5. _____
   _____

6. _____
   _____
   _____

7. _____
   _____
   _____

8. _____
   _____

9. _____
   _____

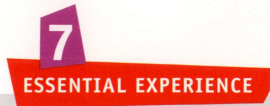

ESSENTIAL EXPERIENCE

Acrylic (Methacrylate) Nail Enhancements Using Forms

In your own words list the steps for applying acrylic nails in the space provided.

1. _____
   _____
   _____
   _____

2. _____
   _____
   _____

3. _____
   _____
   _____

4. _____
   _____
   _____

5. _____
   _____
   _____
   _____
   _____

6. _____
   _____
   _____

7. _____

_____

_____

_____

8. _____

_____

9. _____

_____

_____

_____

_____

10. _____

_____

11. _____

_____

_____

_____

_____

_____

12. _____

_____

_____

13. _____

_____

_____

_____

_____

_____

14. _____
_____
_____
_____
_____

15. _____
16. _____
_____
_____

17. _____
_____
_____
_____

18. _____
_____

19. _____
_____

20. _____
21. _____
_____
_____
_____

22. _____
_____

ESSENTIAL RUBRICS

Rubrics are used in education for organizing and interpreting data gathered from observations of student performance. It is a clearly developed scoring document used to differentiate between levels of development in a specific skill performance or behavior. A rubric is provided in this study guide as a self-assessment tool to aid you in your behavior development.

Rate your performance according to the following scale:

(1) **Development Opportunity:** There is little or no evidence of competency; Assistance is needed; Performance includes multiple errors.

(2) **Fundamental:** There is beginning evidence of competency; Task is completed alone; Performance includes few errors.

(3) **Competent:** There is detailed and consistent evidence of competency; Task is completed alone; Performance includes rare errors.

(4) **Strength:** There is detailed evidence of highly creative, inventive, mature presence of competency.

Space is provided for comments to assist you in improving your performance and achieving a higher rating.

NAIL TIP APPLICATION PROCEDURE

Performance Assessed	1	2	3	4	Improvement Plan
Pre-service sanitation and set up completed					
Performed client consultation					
Washed and sanitized hands					
Removed polish					
Pushed back eponychium					
Removed cuticle tissue					
Buffed nail/removed shine					
Sized tips					
Applied dehydrator					
Applied adhesive					
Slid on tips with stop, rock and hold procedure					
Trimmed nail tip					
Finished blending					
Shaped nails					
Proceeded with desired service					
Post-service cleanup and appointment scheduling completed					

NAIL TIP APPLICATION PROCEDURE

Performance Assessed	1	2	3	4	Improvement Plan
Pre-service sanitation and set up completed					
Performed client consultation					
Washed and sanitized hands					
Removed existing polish					
Cleaned nails					
Pushed back eponychium and removed cuticle					
Removed oily shine					
Applied nail dehydrator					
Applied nail tips if desired					

27-29

ESSENTIAL RUBRICS—CONT'D

NAIL WRAP APPLICATION PROCEDURE

Performance Assessed	1	2	3	4	Improvement Plan
Cut fabric					
Applied fabric adhesive					
Applied fabric					
Trimmed fabric					
Applied wrap resin					
Applied wrap resin accelerator					
Applied second coat of wrap resin					
Applied second coat of wrap resin accelerator					
Shaped and refined nails					
Buffed wrapped nail					
Removed traces of oil					
Applied polish					
Post-service cleanup and appointment scheduling completed					

NO-LIGHT GEL APPLICATION PROCEDURE

Performance Assessed	1	2	3	4	Improvement Plan
Pre-service sanitation and set up completed					
Performed client consultation					
Washed and sanitized hands					
Removed existing polish					
Cleaned fingernails					
Pushed back eponychium; removed cuticle					
Removed oily shine					
Applied nail tips if desired					
Applied nail dehydrator					
Applied no-light gel					
Cured no-light gel with activator					
Applied second coat of no-light gel					
Shaped and refined nails					
Buffed nails					
Applied nail oil					
Applied hand cream and massaged hand and arm					
Cleaned nail enhancements					
Applied nail polish					
Post-service cleanup and appointment scheduling completed					

ESSENTIAL RUBRICS—CONT'D

ACRYLIC NAIL ENHANCEMENTS PROCEDURE

Performance Assessed	1	2	3	4	Improvement Plan
Pre-service sanitation and set up completed					
Performed client consultation					
Washed and sanitized hands					
Cleaned nails; removed existing polish					
Pushed back eponychium and removed cuticle from nail plate					
Removed oily shine form natural nail surface					
Applied nail dehydrator					
Positioned nail form					
Applied nail primer					
Prepared monomer liquid and polymer powder					
Dipped brush into monomer liquid					
Formed product bead					
Placed bead of product					
Shaped free edge					
Placed second bead of product					
Shaped second bead of product					
Applied product bead					
Applied product to remaining nails					
Removed nail forms					
Shaped nail enhancements					
Buffed nail enhancements					
Applied nail oil and hand cream; massaged hand and arm					
Cleaned nail enhancements					
Applied nail polish					
Post-service cleanup and appointment scheduling completed					

ESSENTIAL RUBRICS—CONT'D

ACRYLIC NAIL ENHANCEMENTS OVER TIPS OR NATURAL NAILS PROCEDURE

Performance Assessed	1	2	3	4	Improvement Plan
Pre-service sanitation and set up completed					
Performed client consultation					
Washed and sanitized hands					
Cleaned nails; removed existing polish					
Pushed back eponychium and removed cuticle from nail plate					
Removed oily shine form natural nail surface					
Applied nail dehydrator					
Applied tips if desired					
Applied nail primer					
Prepared acrylic liquid and powder					
Dipped brush into monomer liquid					
Formed product bead					
Placed bead of product on free edge					
Shaped free edge					
Placed second bead of acrylic on free edge					
Shaped second bead of product					
Applied product beads					
Shaped and refined nail enhancement					
Buffed nail enhancement					
Applied nail oil					
Applied hand cream and massage hand and arm					
Cleaned nail enhancements					
Applied nail polish if desired					
Post-service cleanup and appointment scheduling completed					

ESSENTIAL REVIEW

Please answer the following multiple choice questions by circling the correct answer.

1. UV gel enhancements rely on ingredients from the _____ family.
   a) resin
   b) acrylic
   c) wrap
   d) fiberglass

2. UV gels contain _____ , which are liquids.
   a) monomers
   b) polymers
   c) oliogomers
   d) primers

3. Urethane acrylate and urethane methacrylates are used in making
   _____ .
   a) fiberglass wraps
   b) sculptured nails
   c) UV gels
   d) nail tips

4. The step that makes UV gel nail enhancements different from all other nail enhancements is _____ .
   a) soaking
   b) filing
   c) clipping
   d) curing

5. The measure of how much electricity a UV bulb consumes is called
   _____ .
   a) voltage
   b) ohms
   c) amperes
   d) wattage

6. UV gel product is held and spread with _____ .
   a) synthetic brushes
   b) wooden pushers
   c) natural brushes
   d) metal pushers

7. The product used to improve adhesion of UV gels to the natural nail plate is called _____ .
   a) UV gel glue
   b) UV gel paste
   c) UV gel primer
   d) UV gel buffer

8. Using an applicator brush inserted into nail primer to ensure that the nail plate is covered is called _____ .
   a) priming the tip
   b) natural nail preparation
   c) dehydrating the eponychium
   d) conditioning the nail

ESSENTIAL REVIEW   *continued*

9. UV gel #1 is called _____ .
   a) base coat gel
   b) builder gel
   c) primer coat gel
   d) sealer gel

10. When cured UV gels have a tacky surface called a/an _____ .
    a) integumentary layer
    b) aggressive layer
    c) contour layer
    d) inhibition layer

11. What is used to enhance the adhesion of acrylic nails?
    a) dehydrator
    b) primer
    c) initiator
    d) catalyst

12. A process that joins together monomers to create very long polymer chains is called _____ .
    a) rebalancing
    b) molecular reaction
    c) chain reaction
    d) positive reaction

13. Catalysts are added to the _____ and used to control the set or curing time.
    a) powder
    b) liquid
    c) adhesive
    d) dehydrator

14. Benzoyl peroxide is a/an _____ that is added to the powder to start a chain reaction which leads to the creation of long polymer chains.
    a) initiator
    b) dehydrator
    c) catalyst
    d) primer

15. Using the wrong powder with your chosen liquid could result in nails that are _____ .
    a) too thick and cloudy
    b) too thin and cloudy
    c) not properly cured
    d) not ready for polish

16. The amount of monomer and polymer used to create a bead is called the _____ .
    a) product density
    b) product consistency
    c) mixture formula
    d) mix ratio

ESSENTIAL REVIEW *continued*

17. If equal amounts of liquid and powder are used to create a bead, it is called a/an _____ .
   a) wet bead
   b) medium bead
   c) dry bead
   d) oily bead

18. If twice as much liquid is used as powder, the bead is called a _____ .
   a) wet bead
   b) medium bead
   c) dry bead
   d) oily bead

19. Using the proper mixture of powder and liquid ensures proper set and maximum _____ of the nail enhancement.
   a) flexibility
   b) durability
   c) adaptability
   d) resilience

20. If too little powder is used, the nail enhancement can become _____ .
   a) stronger
   b) brittle
   c) discolored
   d) weaker

21. _____ primer is corrosive to the skin and potentially dangerous to the eyes.
   a) alkaline-based
   b) monomer-based
   c) acid-based
   d) alcohol-based

22. The use of dappen dishes to hold acrylic products helps to _____ .
   a) minimize evaporation
   b) maximize evaporation
   c) minimize condensation
   d) maximize condensation

23. For use with acrylic products, the best brushes are composed of _____ .
   a) sable hair
   b) mink hair
   c) synthetic fiber
   d) bristle fiber

24. For nail salon–related applications, gloves made of _____ work best.
   a) nitrile polyester
   b) nitrile polymer
   c) benzoyl polymer
   d) benzoyl monomer

continued

25. Nail enhancements are hard enough to _____ if they make a clicking sound when lightly tapped with a brush handle.
    a) nip and trim
    b) clip and trim
    d) polish and finish
    d) file and shape

26. Nail enhancement that are not properly maintained, have a greater tendency to _____ .
    a) lift and break
    b) split and chip
    c) grow and strengthen
    d) grow slower

27. The method for maintaining the beauty, durability, and longevity of the artificial nail enhancement is known as _____ .
    a) servicing
    b) rebalancing
    c) reconstructing
    d) restructuring

28. Nipping an acrylic nail may perpetuate a lifting problem and can damage the _____ .
    a) nail bed
    b) eponychium
    c) hyponychium
    d) nail plate

29. Odorless products harden more slowly which creates the tacky layer called the _____ .
    a) exhibition layer
    b) assertion layer
    c) inhibition layer
    d) sticky layer

30. _____ in the powder with the brush may be needed with low odor products in order to create the proper mix of powder and liquid.
    a) multiple circular motions
    b) minimal circular motions
    c) a single stroke
    d) multiple vertical dipping

31. When handling nail adhesive, nail technicians should _____ .
    a) wear safety goggles
    b) wear disposable gloves
    c) apply to eponychium
    d) apply to sidewalls

32. The nail tip should cover no more than _____ of the natural nail.
    a) one-third
    b) one-eighth
    c) one-fourth
    d) one-half

ESSENTIAL REVIEW *continued*

33. Natural oil and shine are removed from the nail plate with a/an

_____ .

a) antibacterial soap
b) abrasive
c) adhesive
d) nail wrap

34. Nail tips are attached to the nail plates by using a _____ .

a) cotton-tipped wooden pusher
b) small nail brush
c) stop, rock, and hold procedure
d) stop, rock, and slide procedure

35. Softened nail tips are removed by _____ .

a) rubbing them off
b) nipping them off
c) pulling them off
d) sliding them off

36. A thin, elongated board with a rough surface is called _____ .

a) an abrasive
b) an adhesive
c) a buffer
d) a file

37. Nail-size pieces of cloth or paper that are bonded to the top of the nail plate with nail adhesive are called _____ .

a) repair patches
b) nail wraps
c) no-light gels
d) buffer wraps

38. A piece of fabric cut to completely cover a crack or break in the nail is called

_____ .

a) a repair patch
b) a nail wrap
c) a no-light gel
d) a fiberglass resin

39. A thin, natural material with a tight weave that becomes transparent when adhesive is applied is _____ .

a) linen
b) fiberglass
c) silk
d) paper

40. An implement designed especially for use on nail tips is called a

_____ .

a) nail clipper
b) nail nipper
c) nail cutter
d) tip cutter

ESSENTIAL DISCOVERIES AND ACCOMPLISHMENTS

In the space below, jot some notes about what concepts of this chapter were hardest for you to understand or remember. Imagine finding yourself suddenly in the role of "teacher" and consider what you would tell your "students" about these difficult concepts. Share your Essential Discoveries with some of the other students in your class and ask if they are helpful to them. You may want to revise your notes based on good ideas shared by your peers. Under Accomplishments, list at least three things you have accomplished since your last entry that relate to your career goals.

Discoveries:

_____

_____

_____

_____

_____

_____

_____

_____

_____

_____

Accomplishments:

_____

_____

_____

_____

_____

SEEKING EMPLOYMENT

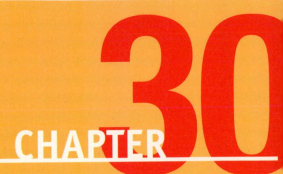

A Motivating Moment: "Success is not measured by what you accomplish but by the opposition you have encountered, and the courage with which you have maintained the struggle against overwhelming odds." —Orison Swett Marden

ESSENTIAL OBJECTIVES

After studying this chapter and completing the Essential Companion components, you should be able to:

1. Discuss the essentials of becoming test-wise.

2. Explain the steps involved in preparing for employment.

3. List and describe the different types of salon businesses.

4. Write an achievement-oriented resume and prepare an employment portfolio.

5. Explain how to explore the job market and research potential employers.

6. Be prepared to complete an effective employment interview.

ESSENTIAL EMPLOYMENT SEEKING

Why do I need to learn about seeking employment while I am still in training?

It's all part of planning your career which is an essential part of planning your life. If you set a goal on the first day of school to become a successful salon owner or a well-known, international platform artist, you must begin your journey toward that goal by obtaining your first career-related position. It's important for you to recognize that when you complete your course of study, your training has really just begun. You have become a student in lifelong learning. Therefore, that first job needs to be suited to your interests, talents, and goals. In addition, it should provide opportunities for your continued growth and professional development. It is not realistic to believe you can obtain your license and find exactly what you are looking for on your first job inquiry. By beginning your search while you are in school, it is far more likely that you will secure an appropriate position upon graduation.

ESSENTIAL CONCEPTS

What do I need to know about seeking employment in order to achieve success in my career?

In addition to developing important personal characteristics such as a positive attitude, desire, and commitment, you will need to identify your talents, skills, and interests to determine the type of salon for which you are best suited. You will learn how to target those salons and observe them in action to confirm whether you want to pursue an employment interview. You must learn to develop an action-oriented resume that will catch the potential employer's eye in a few seconds. You will need to properly prepare for the ever-important job interview. In our society, first impressions matter a great deal. You may have already learned in life that the best qualified applicant does not always get the best job. In fact, the job often goes to the applicant who projects the best image and comes across best during the interview. Thus, learning how to prepare for the interview and how to present yourself during the interview are critical to obtaining the most appropriate position upon graduation.

1

ESSENTIAL EXPERIENCE

Personal Data Page

In preparation for accurate and prompt completion of an employment application, it is beneficial to prepare a personal data page that contains generally the same information. Gather all the necessary information ahead of time and list it on the form provided. It will then be easy to transfer the applicable information to the application form used by your potential employer.

Name _____ Over age 18: _____ Yes _____ No

Address _____

Telephone _____ E-mail _____

Position Desired _____ Date Available _____

Education

High School _____ Graduate: _____ Yes _____ No

Post-secondary _____ Diploma: _____ Yes _____ No

Post-secondary _____ Diploma: _____ Yes _____ No

Post-secondary _____ Diploma: _____ Yes _____ No

Employment History

Where _____ When _____

Position _____ Reason Left _____

Where _____ When _____

Position _____ Reason Left _____

Where _____ When _____

Position _____ Reason Left _____

Significant Skills _____

_____

Awards and Recognitions _____

2

ESSENTIAL EXPERIENCE

Mind Map—The Steps in Seeking Employment

Mind mapping creates a free-flowing outline of material or information. Using the central or key point of seeking employment, diagram the different procedural steps you will need to complete in order to obtain the best possible position. Use terms, pictures, and symbols as desired. Using color will increase your retention of the material. Keep your mind open. Don't worry about where a line or word should go as the organization of the map will usually take care of itself.

3 ESSENTIAL EXPERIENCE

Windowpane—Clinic Achievements

Windowpaning is the process of transferring key elements, points, or steps in a lesson into visual images that are hand sketched into the squares or "panes" of a matrix. Let your mind think in pictures and sketch the essential concepts printed in each of the following windowpanes. Don't be concerned with your artistic ability. Use lines and stick figures to depict the concepts requested for creating an achievement-oriented resume.

Total Regular Clients	Clients Served Weekly	% Clinic in Texture Services
Client Ticket Average	Client Retention Rate	% Clinic in Retail
% Clinic in Haircolor	Attendance Record	Other Accomplishments

4

ESSENTIAL EXPERIENCE

Cover Letter

Using the format describe in your chapter, write a cover letter to accompany your resume when applying for a job.

Date _____

Your Name _____

Your Address _____

City/State _____

Salon Name _____

Salon Address _____

City/State _____

Dear _____ ,

_____

_____

_____

_____

_____

_____

_____

Very cordially yours,

(Signature here)

Your Name
Enclosure

5
ESSENTIAL EXPERIENCE

Interview Preparation

Listed below are several potential questions that may be asked during your interview. Using the space provided, answer the questions to the best of your ability. This exercise will help you be more thoroughly prepared for that important interview.

What did you like best about your training? _____

_____

Are you punctual and regular in attendance? _____

What skills do you feel are your strongest? _____

_____

What skills do you feel are your weakest? _____

_____

Are you a team player? _____ Please explain: _____

_____

Are you flexible? _____ Please explain: _____

_____

What are your career goals? _____

_____

What days/hours are you available to work? _____

Do you have your own transportation? _____

What obstacles, if any, would prevent you from keeping your commitment to

full-time employment? _____

_____

What assets will you bring to the salon and this position? _____

_____

5 ESSENTIAL EXPERIENCE *continued*

Who is the most important person you have met in your work/education experience and why? _____

_____

Explain some strategies you would use in handling a difficult client. _____

_____

How do you feel about retailing? _____

_____

What is your philosophy about attending continuing education programs, seminars, and shows? _____

Are you willing to personally invest in your professional development? _____

_____

Describe ways in which you feel you provide excellent customer service.

_____

_____

Please share some examples of consultation questions you might ask a client.

_____

_____

List steps you would take to build a solid client base and ensure that clients return. _____

_____

ESSENTIAL EXPERIENCE

Word Scramble

Scramble	Correct Word
ticedduve gninsaoer	_ _ _ _ _ _ _ _ _ _ _ _ _ _ _ _ _
	Clue: Used to reach logical conclusions.
loftropoi	_ _ _ _ _ _ _ _ _
	Clue: Collection of documents that reflect your skills.
usemer	_ _ _ _ _ _
	Clue: Summary of education and experience.
krow chiet	_ _ _ _ _ _ _ _ _
	Clue: Commitment to delivering worthy service for value received.
yolpemmten	_ _ _ _ _ _ _ _ _ _
	Clue: Something you pursue upon graduation.
nucomcamiinot	_ _ _ _ _ _ _ _ _ _ _ _ _
	Clue: Something needed to interact effectively with clients.
trigeytin	_ _ _ _ _ _ _ _ _
	Clue: Commitment to a strong code of moral and artistic values.
frenchais	_ _ _ _ _ _ _ _ _
	Clue: Having a national name and image consistent with the organization.
shemtnilbatse	_ _ _ _ _ _ _ _ _ _ _ _ _
	Clue: A place where you may obtain employment.
weevtiinr	_ _ _ _ _ _ _ _ _
	Clue: A meeting where your qualifications are considered.

7

ESSENTIAL EXPERIENCE

Why I Chose Cosmetology

One of the most important tasks you can complete in preparing your professional portfolio and in preparing for an effective interview is writing a brief statement about why you have chosen a career in cosmetology. In the space provided, write such a statement. Remember to include such points as an explanation of what you love about your new career; a description of your philosophy about the importance of teamwork and how you see yourself as a contributing team player; and a description of methods you would employ to increase clinic and retail revenue.

_____

_____

_____

_____

_____

_____

_____

_____

_____

_____

_____

_____

_____

_____

_____

ESSENTIAL REVIEW

Using the following words, fill in the blanks below to form a thorough review of Chapter 30: Seeking Employment. (Please note that the appropriate page(s) in the textbook are referenced, but should not be referred to until you have completed the questions based on your own knowledge.) Words or terms may be used more than once or not at all.

10 seconds	broad	hardest	self-confident
2 minutes	bullheadedness	ideals	self-motivation
20 seconds	career goals	illegal	smiling
20	cheating	integrity	solidified
30	conclusions	legal	speed
50	contacts	motivation	studying
60	course content	multiple choice	test-wise
70	crib notes	negative	timing
80	documents	network	transferable
90	down-time	neutral	true/false
313,000	drawings	portfolio	two million
appropriate	easiest	practice	willpower
assumptions	English	qualifying	work ethic
attention	family member	responsibilities	
autobiography	half million	resume	

1. Top professionals in the field of cosmetology were not born successful; they achieved success with their _____ , energy, and persistence.

2. Of all the factors that will affect your test performance on the licensing examination, the most important is your mastery of _____ .

3. A test-wise student begins to prepare for test-taking by practicing the daily habits and time management that are an important part of effective _____ .

4. On test day, it is a good idea to arrive early with a _____ attitude; be alert, calm, and ready for the challenge.

5. When taking a test, answer the _____ questions first.

6. Deductive reasoning is the process of reaching logical _____ by employing logical reasoning.

ESSENTIAL REVIEW *continued*

7. When applying deductive reasoning in test-taking, watch for "key" words or terms and look for _____ conditions or statements.

8. When taking a _____ test, read the entire question carefully, including all the choices.

9. An effective tip when preparing for the practical examination is to participate in "mock" licensing examinations, including the _____ of applicable examination criteria.

10. Completion of the personal inventory of characteristics and skills helps you identify any areas needing further _____ and determine where to focus the remainder of your training.

11. One key characteristic that will not only help you get the position you want, but will help you keep it is _____ .

12. You have a strong _____ when you believe that work is good and you are committed to delivering worthy service for the value received from your employer.

13. In the United States alone, the professional salon business numbers over _____ establishments that employ more than 1.6 million active cosmetologists.

14. A basic value-priced salon may be a good starting place for a recent graduate because it provides for the practice of many types of haircuts, which increase self-confidence and _____ .

15. A _____ is a written summary of your education and work experience.

16. The average time a potential employer will spend scanning your resume to determine if you should be granted an interview is about _____ .

17. When writing a resume, it is more important to focus on your achievements rather than your _____ .

18. Skills which you have already mastered at other jobs that can be put to use in the new position are known as _____ .

19. An employment portfolio is a collection, usually bound, of photos and _____ that reflect your skills, accomplishments, and abilities in your chosen career field.

ESSENTIAL REVIEW *continued*

20. One way to determine if your portfolio portrays you and your career skills in the most positive light is to run it by a _____ party for feedback and suggestions about how to make it more interesting and accurate.

21. When visiting salons prior to requesting an employment interview, remember that is important to never burn your bridges, but rather build a _____ of contacts who have a favorable opinion of you.

22. _____ is the universal language.

23. On an employment application, questions regarding race, religion, or national origin are considered to be _____ .

24. Make sure your resume focuses on information that is relevant to your _____ goals.

25. Having a complete and thorough knowledge of the subject matter and understanding the strategies for taking tests successfully means that you are _____ .

ESSENTIAL DISCOVERIES AND ACCOMPLISHMENTS

In the space below, jot some notes about what concepts of this chapter were hardest for you to understand or remember. Imagine finding yourself suddenly in the role of "teacher" and consider what you would tell your "students" about these difficult concepts. Share your Essential Discoveries with some of the other students in your class and ask if they are helpful to them. You may want to revise your notes based on good ideas shared by your peers. Under Accomplishments, list at least three things you have accomplished since your last entry that relate to your career goals.

Discoveries:

_____

_____

_____

_____

_____

_____

_____

_____

_____

_____

_____

Accomplishments:

_____

_____

_____

_____

_____

ON THE JOB

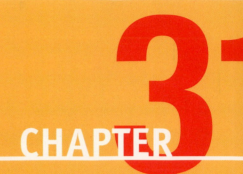

A Motivating Moment: "The place to begin building any relationship is inside ourselves, inside our circle of influence, our own character."—Stephen R. Covey

ESSENTIAL OBJECTIVES

After studying this chapter and completing the Essential Companion components, you should be able to:

1. Describe the qualities that help a new employee succeed in a service profession.

2. List the habits of a good salon team player.

3. Explain the function of a job description.

4. Describe three different ways in which salon professionals are compensated.

5. Create a personal budget.

6. List the principles of selling products and services in the salon.

7. List the most effective ways to build a client base.

ON THE JOB ESSENTIALS

Why do I need to learn about making the transition from school to work?

It has been said that as much as 80% of your career success will result from personal attributes such as your people skills, your ability to communicate, your visual integrity, and your goal orientations. If only 20% of your career success has to do with your technical skills, it stands to reason that there are many more qualities you need to work on to achieve that desired level of success. The cosmetologists who achieve that goal, who stay with the profession longer than the rest, who own or work in successful salons, and enjoy all the rewards of success, all started out with stars in their eyes. However, they knew it took more than just a dream. They knew it would take commitment and hard work and they made sure they were prepared for every opportunity that knocked.

As professionals-in-training they came to school early and stayed late as needed. They accepted those late clients without whining; they wrapped and rewrapped those design texture services on mannequin after mannequin to ensure quality and competitive speed. They read industry journals and stayed abreast of the daily changes happening within the field of cosmetology. The important thing to remember here is that as a professional-in-training, you are about to become a full-fledged, licensed professional.

If you consider yourself among this elite class, you know that you were not born but made yourself who you are today by your own desires and energies and persistence. You recognize that being a stylist is not a 9-to-5 job 4 days a week. It's being there whenever your clients need you. You know that it's going the extra mile, taking the extra client, biting back those angry words that spring up when a client is rude or a coworker is unfair. It's paying your dues, mastering your craft, building self-confidence, and developing strong personal pride in your accomplishments.

ON THE JOB

ESSENTIAL CONCEPTS

What do I need to know about making the transition from school to work in order to maintain satisfaction and success on the job?

While you are probably highly excited about having your first paying job in your new career, there are a number of responsibilities that go along with that paycheck. Your school environment has been a relatively safe and comfortable one. Here, you have had the opportunity to practice service after service to get to the desired results. On the job, your clients will expect the desired results the first time around. In school you have had to deal with the institution's tardy policy, which is probably quite lenient compared to that of a salon. Clients are not very forgiving when you are not at work at the appointed time to provide their service.

While in school you probably had more flexibility in dealing with your personal schedule as it related to your class schedule. On the job you will be expected to be at work every day as scheduled, promptly, and ready to work when you arrive. At school you may have had the opportunity to do your hair or your makeup after you clocked in—not so in the workplace. If you just didn't feel like going to school on any given day, perhaps you just didn't go. A job with a paycheck brings with it an expectation of more maturity than that.

You need to realize that, on the job, you are responsible for many more decisions and for performing in a professional manner at all times, even when you do not feel like it. On the job you will need to be focused on constantly building a business rather than watching the clock to see how long it is until your required hours have been clocked. In addition, you will need to concentrate on furthering your knowledge and skills to remain abreast of all the new trends, tools, and techniques your new job presents. All in all, it's an exciting new opportunity. One that has many rewards accompanied by many responsibilities.

1 ESSENTIAL EXPERIENCE

Evaluate Your Skills—Are You Job Ready?

Take a few minutes to think back over your training and your clinic experience and reflect on all you have learned that you didn't know when you started. Give yourself a hearty pat on the back for your accomplishments. Then evaluate your skills and check those in which you feel confident. If you need more practice, indicate by checking that column. Then make a personal commitment to improve in those areas.

Subject Area	Competent	Need Improvement
Infection control	_____	_____
Product knowledge	_____	_____
Hair chemistry	_____	_____
Shampooing	_____	_____
Haircutting		
Blunt shapes	_____	_____
Graduated shapes	_____	_____
Layered shapes	_____	_____
Clipper cutting	_____	_____
Other cutting techniques	_____	_____
Hair texturizing		
Texture services	_____	_____
Relaxer services	_____	_____
Mixing solutions	_____	_____
Wrapping	_____	_____
Processing	_____	_____
Haircoloring		
Color wheel	_____	_____
Levels of color	_____	_____
Brush application	_____	_____
One process	_____	_____
Two process	_____	_____
Retouch	_____	_____
Foil highlights	_____	_____
Mixing color (tube and liquid)	_____	_____
Style finishing		
Blow-dry	_____	_____
Round brush	_____	_____
Curling iron	_____	_____
Wet sets	_____	_____
Styling aids	_____	_____

ESSENTIAL EXPERIENCE *continued*

Client communications
     Eye contact   ____   ____
     Handshake   ____   ____
     Open-ended questions   ____   ____
     Active listening   ____
     Developing rapport   ____   ____
Client consultation
     Greeting   ____   ____
     Analysis   ____   ____
     Recommendations   ____   ____
Client record keeping   ____   ____
Client development   ____
Client retention   ____   ____
Client referrals   ____   ____
Client rebooking   ____   ____
Retail product sales   ____   ____
Ticket upgrading   ____   ____
Salon/clinic teamwork   ____   ____
Work ethic   ____   ____
Productivity   ____   ____
Receptionist duties   ____
Industry knowledge   ____   ____
Time management   ____   ____
Goal setting   ____   ____
Personal finances   ____   ____
Job hunting skills   ____   ____
Career planning   ____   ____

2 ESSENTIAL EXPERIENCE

Technical Skills Improvement

Based on the analysis you completed in Essential Experience 1, create a plan of action for every area you checked as needing improvement. Record your plan in the space provided.

_____

_____

_____

_____

_____

_____

_____

_____

_____

_____

_____

_____

_____

_____

_____

3

Career Management

In today's market there are more jobs available than there are stylists to fill them. Thus, you owe it to yourself and your potential new employer to find the best fit possible. Once you have made that decision, stick with it and give it your absolute best as long as you can. Job hopping early in your career is not good for your professional development or your reputation. Following are several pointers that will help you right from the start. In the column Plan of Action, explain how you intend to make the most of each suggestion.

Pointer	Plan of Action
Master the techniques you learned in Chapter 30 to ensure you find the right job for your strengths and preferences.	
Understand that your income grows when you work harder, build a sound client base, volunteer for extra clients, sell retail, and show initiative and ambition.	
Arrive for work at least 15 minutes prior to your first client, dressed and groomed, ready to work.	
Have your station set up and ready for each scheduled service before the client arrives.	
Know that your clients and the salon are relying on you to be there. Only call in sick if you are absolutely sick.	
Have realistic expectations of how much money you will earn your first year. It takes time to build a loyal client base.	
Build a realistic personal budget and stick to it. Don't spend more than you make!	
Continue to study, train, and expand your personal and technical skills.	
Join your local cosmetology association and attend meetings faithfully.	

ESSENTIAL EXPERIENCE

Planning Your Future

You are about to complete a major step in your journey toward career success: graduation from cosmetology school. Now it's time to think about building a client base for the future. If you have already targeted area salons and secured a position in one of them, it is appropriate to begin building a client base to join you there.

Create a client development list. These are people you would like to contact about trying your services. Determine how many clients you would like to have when you begin your new job. Create a plan with a goal of contacting a certain number of people every week for at least 1 month. Give these contacts your new place of employment and schedule them for an appointment.

After you get into the salon and perform the services, follow up each salon visit with a phone call and ask about the service you provided. Make sure they are still satisfied and find out if there is anything else you can do for them. If possible, rebook them for a future service.

Use the following space to list the potential clients you want to contact.

Name   **Phone Number**

_____

_____

_____

_____

_____

_____

_____

_____

_____

ESSENTIAL EXPERIENCE

Teamwork

As a contributing team member in the salon, you will be called upon to deal with a variety of problems or situations on a regular basis. In order to build your teamwork skills while you are in school, work with a couple of other classmates. Consider the following situations and how you would handle them in the workplace. Record your results in the space provided.

1. You each arrive for work with a fully booked schedule for the day. The manager and two other stylists have been stricken with the flu and will not make it into work today. You and your teammates have to decide how to handle the clients of the other three stylists. What do you do?

   _____

   _____

   _____

2. Your salon owner is remodeling the facility, which includes reorganizing the space and assigning new work stations to everyone. You and your classmates are to discuss and develop some criteria the owner could use in assigning new stations because some spaces are more desirable than others.

   _____

   _____

   _____

3. The salon's manager states the plan of implementing a retail bonus plan for all stylists and asks for your help in developing the policy. You and your classmates are to create a retail bonus plan that you would recommend for adoption.

   _____

   _____

   _____

6 ESSENTIAL EXPERIENCE

The Job Description

Assume the role of owner of a highly successful salon. Write a job description for a junior stylist, listing all the factors you deem appropriate to the position.

_____

_____

_____

_____

_____

_____

_____

_____

_____

_____

_____

_____

_____

_____

_____

_____

_____

_____

_____

ESSENTIAL REVIEW

Using the following words, fill in the blanks below to form a thorough review of Chapter 31: On The Job. Words may be used more than once or not at all.

client	doubt	increasing	serving
client	feelings or desires	job description	temptation
consultations	financial	mathematical	ticket upgrading
commissions	grateful	respectful	transition
compensation	hourly	retailing	
conflict	immature	salon	

1. When you become the employee of a salon, you will be expected to put the needs of the _____ and _____ ahead of your own.

2. Making the _____ from school to work can be difficult.

3. The number one thing to remember when you are in a service business is that your work revolves around _____ your clients.

4. In the salon you will have to quickly get used to putting your own _____ aside and putting the needs of the salon and the client first.

5. Getting to work on time is _____ not only to your clients but also to your coworkers who will have to handle your clients if you are late.

6. Remember that it is an honor to have a job that will provide you and your family with financial stability, so be very _____ .

7. Although you may not like or agree with the salon manager or her rules, you must give her the benefit of the _____ .

8. Thinking that you will never need to learn anything more once you are out of school is _____ and limiting.

9. Given the stress of a typical salon, there will be lots of opportunities for you to become negative or to have conflicts with your teammates. Resist the _____ to give in to maliciousness and gossip.

10. The most difficult part of being in a relationship, whether it is a personal or professional relationship, is when _____ arises.

11. When assuming a new position, you are agreeing to do everything as it is written down in a _____ , so if you are unclear about something or need more information, it is your responsibility to ask.

12. Being paid an _____ rate is usually the best way for new salon professionals to start out.

13. _____ are paid on percentages of your total service dollars and can range anywhere from 25% to 60%, depending on your length of time at the salon and your performance levels.

14. When deciding whether a certain _____ method is right for you, it is important to be aware of what your monthly expenses are and to have a personal financial budget and plan in place.

15. Ask a senior stylist to sit in on one of your _____ and to make note of areas where you can improve.

16. Although a career in the beauty industry is very artistic and creative, it is also a career that requires _____ understanding and planning.

17. Many people are afraid of the word "budget" because they think it will be too restrictive on their spending or because they think they need to be _____ geniuses in order to work with a budget.

18. You will want to think about other ways to increase your income, including spending less money and _____ service prices.

19. _____ or up-selling services is the practice of recommending and selling additional services to your clients, which may be performed by you or by other practitioners in the salon.

20. _____ is the act of recommending and selling products to your clients for at-home hair, skin, and nail care.

ESSENTIAL DISCOVERIES AND ACCOMPLISHMENTS

In the space below, jot some notes about what concepts of this chapter were hardest for you to understand or remember. Imagine finding yourself suddenly in the role of "teacher" and consider what you would tell your "students" about these difficult concepts. Share your Essential Discoveries with some of the other students in your class and ask if they are helpful to them. You may want to revise your notes based on good ideas shared by your peers. Under Accomplishments, list at least three things you have accomplished since your last entry that relate to your career goals.

Discoveries:

_____

_____

_____

_____

_____

_____

_____

_____

_____

_____

Accomplishments:

_____

_____

_____

_____

_____

THE SALON BUSINESS

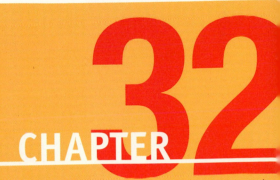

A Motivating Moment: "*If you will call your troubles experiences, and remember that every experience develops some latent force within you, you will grow vigorous and happy, however adverse your circumstances may seem to be.*"
—John Homer Miller

ESSENTIAL OBJECTIVES

After studying this chapter and completing the Essential Companion components, you should be able to:

1. List the two ways in which you may go into business for yourself.

2. List the factors to consider when opening a salon.

3. Name and describe the types of ownership under which a salon may operate.

4. Explain the importance of keeping accurate business records.

5. Discuss the importance of the reception area to a salon's success.

6. Demonstrate good salon telephone techniques.

7. List the most effective forms of salon advertising.

Is the knowledge of business really so important to someone who just wants to be a hair designer?

Absolutely! Even if you never own your own salon, you need to understand the key principles of building and operating a business to ensure your own success. Most individuals entering this exciting field dream of owning their own salon one day. The fact is that more than a few of those graduates actually turn that dream into reality. The more you know about managing and operating an efficient business, the more valuable you become to your future employers.

ESSENTIAL CONCEPTS

What do I need to know about the salon business in order to be successful?

There are many factors to consider before taking the step into ownership or even management. A knowledge of business principles, bookkeeping, business laws, insurance, salesmanship, and psychology is crucial for the successful salon owner or manager. Serving people is one thing; managing people is quite another. Just knowing about business is not enough. You need to develop leadership, self-control, and sensitivity. This whole area of business calls for planning, supervision, control, evaluation, and, above all, teamwork.

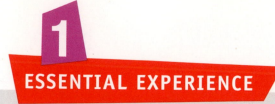

ESSENTIAL EXPERIENCE

Salon Research

Research at least five salons in the area where you may want to work. Your mission is to determine which salon is most suited to your needs. Rate each category on a scale of 1 to 10, with 10 being considered the best. Explain your rating. Use the chart below to track your findings.

Category	Salon 1	Salon 2	Salon 3	Salon 4	Salon 5
Location/Active Business Nearby					
Demographics/Income Area					
Adequate Parking					
Direct Competition Nearby					
Exterior Appearance and Design (attractive)					
Interior Appearance and Design (attractive and efficient)					
Retail Sales Awareness					

2 ESSENTIAL EXPERIENCE

Matching—Regulations, Business Law, and Insurance

Match each of the following essential terms with its definition.

_____ Local regulations

_____ Federal law

_____ State law

_____ Income tax law

_____ Insurance

1. Covers sales taxes, licenses, and employee compensation.

2. Covered by both state and federal government.

3. Covers building renovations.

4. Cover malpractice, premises liability, fire, burglary and theft, and business interruption.

5. Covers Social Security, unemployment compensation, cosmetics and luxury taxes, and OSHA.

3 ESSENTIAL EXPERIENCE

Income and Expense

Assume the following facts:

- Your monthly revenue goal is $10,000.
- The ticket average in your salon is $20.00 per client.
- Your salon is open 5 days per week or an average of 22 days per month.

Based on the above information, determine how many clients you will have to serve per day and how many stylists you will have to employee to reach your revenue goal.

_____

_____

Once you have obtained the above information, apply the percentages taken from the budget on page 660 of your text to the $10,000 gross revenue to determine what your salon profit will be for the month.

Salaries:	$10,000 × 53.5%	=	$ _____
Rent:	$10,000 × 13%	=	$ _____
Supplies:	$10,000 × 5%	=	$ _____
Advertising:	$10,000 × 3%	=	$ _____
Depreciation:	$10,000 × 3%	=	$ _____
Laundry:	$10,000 × 1%	=	$ _____
Cleaning:	$10,000 × 1%	=	$ _____
Utilities:	$10,000 × 1%	=	$ _____
Repairs:	$10,000 × 1.5%	=	$ _____
Insurance:	$10,000 × .75%	=	$ _____
Telephone:	$10,000 × .75%	=	$ _____
Miscellaneous:	$10,000 × 1.5%	=	$ _____
	Total Expenses:		$ _____
	Net Profit:		$ _____

Now, consider what would happen if you were unable stay within the recommended guidelines of your budget. Perhaps your rent is more than the above amount. Maybe you are having to pay more for a cleaning crew or you have several telephone lines and your telephone bill runs around $300 per month. It's important to consider all these factors when setting up a business because the only way to make more money is to increase revenue or reduce expenses or a combination of both.

4

ESSENTIAL EXPERIENCE

Daily Revenue Report Form

On a separate sheet of paper, design a form on which you would track your clients on a daily basis. The form would record their services, retail sales, total sales, and possibly other items as well. You might want to track how the client heard about your salon or other data that would help you analyze your business.

5

ESSENTIAL EXPERIENCE

Job Descriptions

On a separate sheet(s) of paper, write a position description for a stylist and a receptionist in your salon. Be thorough and specific. Outline their general responsibilities as well as their specific duties.

Advertising

In the space provided, design a 3" × 5" newspaper ad for your salon.

In the space provided, write a 30-second radio ad promoting your salon and its services.

_____

_____

_____

_____

_____

_____

_____

Crossword Puzzle

Word	Clue
_____	Should be 3% of your gross income.
_____	Supplies used in the daily business operations.
_____	Ownership is shared by stockholders.
_____	Must understand all provisions that pertain to the landlord and tenant.
_____	Ownership is shared by two or more people.
_____	Largest expense in the salon.
_____	Advertising that allows for close contact with the potential client.
_____	The quarterback of the salon.
_____	Proprietor is owner and manager.
_____	Supplies sold to the client.
_____	Complaints are often handled on this.

7 ESSENTIAL EXPERIENCE *continued*

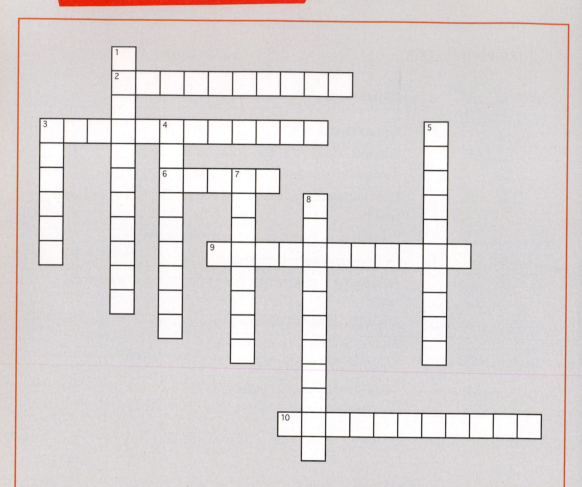

Clues:

Across

2. Advertising that allows for close contact with the potential client
3. The quarterback of the salon
6. Must understand all provisions that pertain to the landlord and tenant
9. Ownership is shared by two or more people
10. Ownership is shared by stockholders

Down

1. Should be 3 percent of your gross income
3. Supplies sold to the client
4. Complaints are often handled on this
5. Proprietor is owner and manager
7. Largest expense in the salon
8. Supplies used in the daily business operations

8
ESSENTIAL EXPERIENCE

Interviewing Personnel

Select a partner and role-play interviewing that person for employment in your salon. Prepare in advance a list of questions you wish to ask him or her. List the questions and his or her responses below.

_____

_____

_____

_____

_____

_____

_____

_____

_____

_____

_____

_____

_____

ESSENTIAL REVIEW

Using the following words, fill in the blanks below to form a thorough review of Chapter 32: The Salon Business. Words or terms may be used more than once or not at all.

advertising	correct grammar	indispensable	equal
consumption	quarterback	investment capital	sole proprietorship
supplies	nerve center	excellent customer	location
retail	overall attitude	service	booth rental
incoming phone	capital	quality inventory	health
calls	business plan	non-compete	
tact	mortgage	agreement	

1. Supplies used in daily business operations are called _____ .

2. An important aspect of the salon's financial success revolves around _____ sales.

3. A satisfied client is the very best form of _____ .

4. The lifeline of the salon is _____ .

5. When handling complaints by phone, respond with self-control, _____ , and courtesy.

6. When using the telephone, you should have a pleasant voice, speak clearly, and use _____ .

7. A well-trained receptionist has been referred to as the _____ of the salon.

8. The reception area of the salon has been referred to as the _____ of the salon.

9. When interviewing potential employees, consider their level of skill, personal grooming, communication skills, and _____ .

10. Money needed to start a new business is known as _____ .

11. In a successful business, a good accountant and an accounting system are _____ .

12. Smooth business management depends on many factors, including sufficient _____ .

ESSENTIAL REVIEW *continued*

13. Another factor that is critical in a successful business is the delivery of
    _____ .

14. If purchasing an existing salon from another individual, it is imperative for
    the agreement to include a _____ .

15. In a partnership, ownership is not necessarily _____ .

16. When the salon is owned by a single individual, who is most often the
    manager, it is known as a _____ .

17. A written description of your business as you see it today or foresee it in
    the next 5 years is known as a _____ .

18. One of the most important factors to consider when planning the success
    of your salon is _____ .

19. _____ is a desirable situation for many practitioners who
    have many steady clienteles and do not have to rely on the salon to stay
    busy.

20. Among the many obligations of a booth renter are: keeping records,
    paying taxes, maintaining inventory, advertising, and carrying adequate
    malpractice and _____ insurance.

ESSENTIAL DISCOVERIES AND ACCOMPLISHMENTS

In the space below, jot some notes about what concepts of this chapter were hardest for you to understand or remember. Imagine finding yourself suddenly in the role of "teacher" and consider what you would tell your "students" about these difficult concepts. Share your Essential Discoveries with some of the other students in your class and ask if they are helpful to them. You may want to revise your notes based on good ideas shared by your peers. Under Accomplishments, list at least three things you have accomplished since your last entry that relate to your career goals.

Discoveries:

_____

_____

_____

_____

_____

_____

_____

_____

_____

_____

Accomplishments:

_____

_____

_____

_____

_____